KEVIN KENDALL

When the Solution is the Problem

From complexity to clarity: a personal journey to overcome serious illness

The only power you have against the
state is the power to not require it's
services...

Contents

Acknowledgement

I wish to thank my family for putting up with me, always being there through difficult times, and not judging me too harshly for my inability to accept my reality.

Also, a special mention for Kathy Aitken, whose input helped turn this book from a series of disjointed ramblings into something coherent and readable.

1

First Things First

There are two ways of learning things. One is through direct experience, and when you learn this way the lessons kind of stick. The other is through passed-on information, which is how we generally acquire the majority of our knowledge – by watching, reading, listening, copying, and most importantly, remembering.

Direct experience led me to write this book. I didn't just read about what I am going to discuss, do not have a formal education in the subject, and never took any tests or exams. As such, I don't have a relevant qualification to help prove my case, am not able to name-drop any famous authors or any renowned academics, and will not be providing a long list of references to peer-reviewed papers supporting my findings. I did decide to try and rectify this before I began writing, so set out to find some officially clever information.

However, I didn't start by looking for scientific research papers. This is because I'm going to tell you a story about how science doesn't always live up to its promises. I will provide references to one or two relevant papers as I go through the book, but for the most part, I am not going to rely on something that, in my case at least, has fallen short of the mark.

Science aside, my first thoughts were that I might be able to find some sort of archetypal reference to what I'm going to focus on, which involves solutions to problems that cause the very problem they are supposed to be solving, but could only find the concept of "fixes that fail", on a very boring website about business strategy. This wasn't exactly what I was looking for because it is concerned with the effect of quick fixes creating additional problems. While I certainly can apply such scenarios to myself, I'm more interested in the idea of a closed loop, where the original problem only exists, or maybe more accurately, persists, because of the solution implemented to fix it.

So I started trawling through some mythology, to see if any tales of old had something in them, but gave up very quickly, even though I believe somewhere in the back of my mind that it would be interesting to learn all about myths and legends from various cultures and different points in history. Maybe this isn't the case at all for me, as while I'd very much like to know all about mythology, this is in the same way I'd like to be able to play a guitar. While I do want to be proficient in such things, I don't have enough desire or motivation to put the required time and effort into doing the actual learning.

I thought psychology might have some answers, and maybe it does somewhere. The basic principles certainly do, but in terms of bigger and more complete concepts and theories, I drew a blank. The internet seemed to want me to understand that psychology offers actual solutions to real or imagined problems, so I moved on.

Next, I thought philosophy might be what I was looking for, but a wall of boredom quickly built itself up in my mind and prevented me from going any further. Perhaps I started with the wrong sort of philosophy or something, but whether this was the case or not, I decided to end that line of investigation. As with mythology and musical instruments, I think my interest in philosophy hovers somewhere around the sound bite level.

I didn't bother with religion, as the basic premise of all religions is that they provide solutions, with those solutions being beyond reproach, so they are unlikely to focus on something causing the very problem it is offering to solve.

I'm not trying to belittle any of these areas of knowledge or belief by telling you this. It is just that I already know what I will be writing about, so it makes no real difference to me whether or not someone else can confirm it, and I have no particular need to learn about it second-hand. Also, my very cursory skim of online search results and a few subsequent websites took me only a few hours, so I will admit straight away that I might not have come up with a whole new perspective on the workings of the world.

However, I have managed to turn my little lot around, in direct contradiction to the advice of many highly qualified experts, who tell me such a thing is not possible. This has taken me the best part of forty years, which, in contrast to the half-hearted search for information I've just described, has provided me with vast amounts of time in the field. Sometimes being in a field often turns out much more illuminating than simply looking at the field, or even just reading and remembering someone else's interpretation of what they think is in the field.

As I said at the start, the thing with acquiring knowledge through direct experience is that once you've got it, it's permanent. Good or bad, useful or not, it doesn't matter. You just know it, and no amount of being told otherwise makes any difference at all.

Rather than waffling on about what I did and what I didn't do concerning things that I'm mostly not going to be writing about, I'll get straight to it.

OK then, I have had the joy of living most of my life with Crohn's Disease, which is the kind of condition nobody wants to talk about. It doesn't grab headlines like more media-friendly illnesses do. While it does have charities and support groups, none of which I have ever had any interaction with, by the way, these groups don't seem able to spread any sort of message about Crohn's to wider society. It is a disease centred on embarrassing things, the kind of things we are taught from an early age to not discuss, namely sickness (the regurgitating of food kind of sickness in addition to the extreme unwellness type), diarrhoea, and eating disorders. Even the name is a bit awkward, so there's not a lot going for it. That being said, it is a truly awful and life-changing condition. The first thing you are supposed to learn when you receive a diagnosis of Crohn's is that there is no cure, meaning you are stuck with it for life. This is something I have never accepted, and will never accept, as to do so implies to me that at some level I must become the disease, which means restrictions and reduced freedom of choice.

I haven't made things easy on myself with my refusal to accept my situation, and have possibly even made it much worse than it might have otherwise been. I also know that adopting such a position puts me at odds with the entire focus of the medical industry. However, it is one of the few things in life where I have consistently been willing to cut off my nose to spite my face. The upshot of my never-ending stubbornness is that I have finally managed to reverse my ill health. At fifty years old, I am reasonably healthy by any measure, impossibly so if my background is taken into account. I don't need any medication or any other kind of therapy and don't have to plan my nutrition or day-to-day existence with absolute precision. I can get on with life as a normal person. This is in direct contrast to the very bleak existence I was facing just a few short years ago.

To make these positive improvements, the steps I have taken are very specific and incredibly simple. As such I think I may have something of real value to share with others, and this is what led me to write it down. You might be wondering why I need to write an entire book if it is as simple as I am saying. While it is true that I could fit what I need to say in a pamphlet, or even on a single sheet of paper in bullet point format, it is also true you probably wouldn't believe what I have to say if that was all I did.

The overall strategy I have adopted directly contradicts most of what every interested party has to say about a disease such as mine, and by interested party I mean health professionals, research scientists, the pharmaceutical industry, specialists in food and nutrition, support groups and charities, the government, the holistic healing industry, friends and family, and perhaps most importantly, until very recently, myself. So I'm going to have to convince you that I am right, and since I'm unwilling to trudge through science and academia, I'm going to have to show you how I came to the understanding I finally arrived at, after several decades of getting nowhere.

In this book, I'm going to start with a bit of background about how my disease came about, then stayed about, and then got worse as time went on. This is to give you some context as to just how bad an illness Crohn's can be, but also to show how my perception of the world gradually changed, something that was essential to resolving my predicament. I'll then explain how I have reversed my situation, including the specific steps I have taken, along with my reasoning behind them. This includes why I am convinced that the medical treatments for Crohn's can only ever create more of the disease they are supposed to be treating.

I will also point out right now, that I am not selling you anything beyond this book – it is not leading into a product, or towards any kind of additional course or seminar. Everything I have to offer you is contained within these pages. But enough of that for now, let's begin with what I am certain was the single biggest defining part of my trajectory towards being someone with a lifelong and extremely debilitating illness...

2

A Day I'll Never Forget

There's never an absolute starting point, because everything is always the result of something else, but I'll start with me at the age of twelve, back in the first half of 1986. Up to then I had always excelled academically, was fit, healthy, reasonably good at sports, and could carry off the appearance of being an almost normal child. Well, sort of almost normal, anyway.

I had a very good memory, which was great for sailing through schoolwork, but also meant I remembered every single thing I had either said or done wrong, so I had a wealth of background data to beat myself up with psychologically. I had been a very picky eater for as long as I could remember, so my diet wasn't particularly broad and probably not very nutritious, but I had plenty of energy and seemed to get by. Being good at learning, I had become a true believer in science and the modern world, so was looking forward to things like holidays in space, which were on the brink of becoming reality and would be ready to take bookings by the time I was all grown up.

Also, work was soon to become a thing of the past, and clean, free energy via nuclear fusion was just about ready to take care of all the world's electricity requirements. Today, almost forty years later, nuclear fusion remains at the same point of being almost ready, which is worth taking note of. Just like holiday tours of the solar system.

I even managed to attach a positive spin to the impending doom of global warming, which was also gathering momentum at the time, in stark contrast to the impending doom of global cooling which had been on the brink of happening just ten years earlier. Now that warming was the thing to worry about, the ice caps were going to melt, and the sea levels were going to rise. This meant I would live closer to the sea, so it wouldn't be as far to travel to go sailing in my yacht, the one I was going to own to pass the time, since I wouldn't have to work and would probably not be exploring outer space all the time.

I also didn't have to worry about health because disease was soon to be a thing of the past, and at any rate, medicine could fix anything in the modern, space-age world that was supposedly coming into focus.

Aside from all these alleged leaps forward into the future, in the UK in the 1980s, there still was a mass vaccination drive against tuberculosis, so when children were around twelve years old, people in white coats came to school and gave the whole year group a BCG vaccine (Bacillus Calmette–Guérin - Bacillus is a genus of bacteria and Calmette–Guérin are the names of the inventors of the injection).

Back then, the UK still operated within a fairly socialist mindset. It still does to an extent, but this was more apparent 40 years ago. It had come about after the Second World War, with so-called cradle-to-grave social care and welfare policies. Not full-on communism or anything, but a sort of mostly capitalist society mixed with a safety net of state intervention for the old, the ill, and the unemployed people. The origins of that probably had something to do with the country needing to repopulate and rebuild itself after the war, and likely had very little to do with the ruling classes suddenly developing any love for the peasants, but that's another story. Things were changing rapidly, thanks (on the surface at least) to the policies of the Conservative Party under the leadership of Margaret Thatcher, but it still seemed entirely normal to expect the state to provide.

Speaking from my perspective at the time, it seemed barbaric that in other countries people had to pay for things such as healthcare by themselves. I have a feeling that most British people thought similarly and that most still do, but you'd have to go and ask them to confirm this. I still do think healthcare should be free because the need for it tends to go hand-in-hand with a lack of ability to pay, but where I probably differ from many British people is in having finally acknowledged that placing your health into the hands of other people has replaced one set of problems with a whole range of different ones. One of these is the fact that various people stand to profit from your ill health.

Back to where I am going with this, the beliefs that Britain had installed in its population for many years meant most of us didn't question things like people in white coats turning up and injecting stuff into you. The experts knew what they were doing, after all. If they said you needed a jab for something, you went along and got your jab, and therein lies one of the fundamental flaws of such a mindset. It is all well and good if the people making the decisions are making the right decisions. Even if one assumes they are, something that can never always be the case, there are always going to be some individuals who will suffer as a result. It then becomes a game of numbers and ideas like 'the greater good' come into existence, a concept that seems perfectly acceptable, at least until you find yourself on the wrong side of the equation.

There would have been people who asked questions, but the prevailing attitude of the majority of those going through the state-run education system was that you stand in line, roll up your sleeve, and get your medicine.

I still clearly remember the vaccination day. It became a test of character – an opportunity to prove oneself by not showing any signs of distress or weakness. If you could manage a smile on your way out of the jab room past the queue still waiting to go in, then all the better.

I remember a feeling of dread leading up to this. I didn't want to get my shot but couldn't risk being seen as soft (a bit of a pointless exercise since my peers already thought I was anyway), so I never said I wanted to give it a miss, even though there wasn't anyone to say this to if I had plucked up the courage to do so.

The day of the injections came, and I dutifully joined the queue when my class was called. It turned out that the stories of pain and suffering trickling down from older year groups were not entirely unfounded. On the way back to class I still managed to show my strength of character though, smiling when I thought anyone was looking, even though my arm felt like it had just been hit with a sledgehammer. I even managed a chuckle when I saw one of my classmates sitting on a chair outside, pale as a sheet, and on the verge of passing out. At least I wasn't that pathetic...

Back in class, which was a German lesson with a teacher called Mr Giles, I resumed my studies. It was something about Hans and his family.

"Ich habe einen VW" (pronounced *vey-vow*) is one of the few things I remember from German and is entirely irrelevant to this slice of my story. However, should my life ever depend on telling a native German speaker that I am the owner of a Volkswagen then I've got that covered.

In the classroom, the desks were arranged in a double U formation, one outside of the other, with the blackboard and teacher's desk at the open end of the U's. My seat was about halfway down the inner U of desks, so I was facing the children sitting on the other side of it, a few feet away.

After a few minutes, I began to feel a bit queasy and more than a little lightheaded, then started producing a lot of horrible, cold, clammy sweat. The ordeal wasn't quite over yet, I concluded, so I tried to focus, thinking the worst thing that could happen would be me sitting on a chair outside showing all my lack of character to everyone in the school. I managed to hold it together for maybe a few seconds, then realised I was going to throw up. Like the good little cog in the machine I had learned to be, I put my hand up to ask if I could go to the toilet, but never got to ask. A stream of pink projectile vomit suddenly spewed forth from my mouth, travelling as far as the desks opposite. It was like something out of the film *The Exorcist*, although I was still several years away from seeing that film, so wasn't able to draw such an analogy at the time. I promptly passed out for a few moments, then came around and managed to produce another equally forceful stream of vomit.

At that point I wasn't feeling too good, to say the least, and to this day I still remember being most surprised at the next set of events. This is in no immediately obvious way connected to the general idea I want to convey in this book, just like being able to confirm ownership of a VW in German isn't, but I'm still somewhat perplexed by it, so I'm going to tell you anyway, in more detail than I probably need to, which if the truth is told, is no detail at all. Before I get to what happened, what should have happened is something along the lines of this...

The teacher, having been fully briefed about the potential of a serious reaction to the medical procedure that had been administered just minutes earlier to one of the children in his care, should have immediately recognised such a reaction in one of those children, and should then have gone to get the medical crash team into the classroom (he would have had to go to get them since mobile phones were still a few years away so he couldn't have simply called or texted them). This is the crash team that should have been on standby to deal with potentially life-threatening incidents, the kind that might occur when injecting an entire year group of children with some concoction of unspecified origin. The crash team, having been fully trained concerning said reactions, would have an antidote to the medicine in question, and would administer it forthwith to any child in the midst of such a reaction, to prevent negative health consequences from ensuing. However, nothing of the sort happened – the reality was more like this...

The children sitting opposite me weren't best pleased when I ejected a stream of Exorcist-style vomit over them. So their cries of disgust and distress were entirely understandable. The teacher's reaction I still find less so. Rather than showing any concern whatsoever, he flew off the handle and gave me a good telling-off.

"How dare you be sick over my classroom! Get this mess cleaned up, right now!"

I was fighting to stay conscious at that moment, but he was

shouting at me to start cleaning! I'm not sure how I was going to achieve such a goal even if I could have stood up, as I wasn't privy to the whereabouts of the required cleaning equipment, such as mops and buckets, but that didn't matter, I was supposed to get the room cleaned. There was no crash team, since the injections were perfectly good and safe, and were fine to give out with no medical backup whatsoever.

I didn't clean anything up in the end. I know that much, but I don't know who did and I can't remember anything else about the rest of that particular day.

The next day I felt a bit better, aside from having become something of a laughingstock around school. It was bad enough thinking that I would have to live with this embarrassment, but other than that I thought it was over. Being a great new reference point for me to remind myself of my general unworthiness, rather than begin to ponder on what had happened, I managed to blame myself and my intrinsic weakness as a human being for not being able to handle a little injection. Thus my belief in the state and the infallibility of science wasn't affected in the slightest.

Things seemed to return to normal over the next couple of weeks. I was off my food a bit, but this wasn't entirely out of the ordinary. I just didn't feel hungry and then felt full quite quickly when I did eat. I started getting odd little pains in my stomach from time to time, but these would go away, so I didn't think to worry about them.

Over the next few months, I continued not wanting to eat much on a more ongoing basis and started losing some weight as a result. The pains kept coming and going, but every time I experienced pain I perceived it as an isolated incident, so didn't start building up any true picture of what was gathering in the background. I remember a couple of times when classmates told me that my face had a strange colour to it. Since this was a state-run comprehensive school, we hadn't learned about the usage of descriptive words like 'pallid', so the comments were along the lines of, "Here, your face is f**kin' green."

The BCG jabs had been sometime in February, and apart from the green face thing, the stomach pains, the increasing lack of appetite, and the weight loss, life remained fairly normal for a time. Obviously, with the benefit of hindsight, there was nothing normal about what I was experiencing, but one of the main things you learn at school is how to put on a front to hide your insecurities and weaknesses. That's probably the main lesson imparted by school, to make people ready for the world of work, where it becomes a prerequisite to fake an interest in repeating the same mind-numbing tasks all day long, with interludes to discuss graphs and spreadsheets full of pointless information, and repeating it all five days a week until you are old enough to retire and die. Having already been through several years of this 'education' I was reasonably good at avoiding or suppressing the issues I was facing and was able to pretend to myself and everyone else that everything was OK.

I couldn't hide it for long though. By the summer, I was struggling considerably with PE, the abbreviation for physical education classes. This was back when being educated physically was thought best achieved by the school employing bullies to terrorise children into compliance, along the lines of an army boot camp. Having always been reasonably good at sports I had, up to that point, avoided the attention of the PE teachers for the most part. I always felt sorry for the people who simply weren't any good (meaning the handful of fat kids and geeks who existed back then). The PE teachers were merciless, shouting and screaming at them for no good reason, then throwing the ball of whatever game we were playing at their faces.

Just as an aside, the catchphrase of one of my PE teachers is burned into my memory forever. Mr Holmes would pull people into line with the words, "Sit doon yer cloon before a' knock yer doon!" I have to provide that phrase in his original accent because it doesn't work the same in Queen's English. Perhaps I should say King's English now we have a King and not a Queen, but I'm not sure of the finer points of such etiquette. Whatever it is, it's a term British people use to describe correct use of the English language. So the translation in proper English would read, "Sit down you clown before I knock you down," but this does not offer the same scope for the vehemence he managed to apply to the words.

I grew up around Newcastle in the Northeast of England, where we have a very distinctive accent, known as Geordie. Mr Holmes' voice was only partially Geordie though, mixed with elements from somewhere else, maybe Sunderland, or perhaps even Cumbria or Yorkshire, so unlike a proper Geordie, he drew out the 'doon', 'cloon', and especially the final 'doon', just before whatever ball he had hold of went flying towards whoever had incurred his wrath. As far as I remember, he never managed to get a fat kid to lose weight and never managed to imbue an uncoordinated geek with any athletic prowess via his methods, but he never gave up trying.

As I mentioned just before digressing, I had always been somewhere in the middle of the sporting hierarchy, so managed to get by mostly unnoticed. Confidence held me back rather than a lack of coordination or an unhealthy physical condition. However, by the summer of 1986, I was finding myself out of breath very quickly, and my abilities fell off rapidly. This was the point where I started thinking there might be something wrong with me. Since it was several months after the BCG injection, and since I had managed to successfully not pay any attention to the earlier warning signs, I still did not make any connection between the vaccination and the health crisis I was now beginning to feel. I did get to experience some of the negative attention of the PE teachers, who in their wisdom, decided I simply wasn't trying hard enough anymore and told me in no uncertain terms to buck my ideas up.

"But sir, I'm not feeling very well at all, and am starting to look like I'm quite literally dying in front of you," was considered a very poor excuse, such is the importance of sporting prowess. After all, where would civilisation be if every child wasn't adept at running up and down a field after some kind of ball?

Then the summer holidays came. In the UK we got, and school children still get, a six-week holiday for the summer. The roots of this long holiday go back to harvest time when every available pair of hands was required to bring in the crops, and it has remained in place to this day. Today it is mostly due to teachers needing the full six weeks to go on extended middle-class adventures, doing things like towing caravans around Europe, unlike most other people who are lucky to get one or maybe two weeks off work.

Back to my story, it was soon September, and with that came the start of a new school year. I was starting to feel very unwell by this point, losing weight rapidly, not being able to hold much food down, looking very pale, still getting stomach pains but more consistently and more severely now, being sick (as in the spewing up usage of the word sick – I probably should use the word 'vomit' rather than 'sick' because 'sick' covers a wide range of possibilities, but 'vomit' has always seemed a bit too posh a way of saying it to me), and I was starting to struggle enormously with my energy levels. After a few months of going back and forwards to the doctors, and being told there was nothing wrong, they finally did some investigations and found that I had an ulcer in my duodenum (the bit where the stomach drains out to the small bowel). This was blocking the exit to my stomach(*), hence the inability to eat and all the other problems. The vaccination from months earlier was now an item of history, so any chance of forming a link had disappeared. I was given some ulcer medication (Ranitidine), sent on my way, and told I would get better soon.

*Later in the book I will explain a bit more about ulcers and inflammation, which will help illustrate how an ulcer, according to the actual definition of what one is, is not technically the thing causing the blockage. However, I was presented with the diagnosis of 'an ulcer causing a blockage' at the time.

Something I find strange about all of this is that there was no consideration of why a thirteen-year-old child might have a stomach ulcer (my birthday is in June so I was a year older in terms of numbers from when I started this chapter). The medical system seems, to me anyway, to not do anything at all to find the roots of an illness, especially one somewhat peculiar, to say the least, in someone so young. It's not like I'd been drinking and smoking and partying to excess at that point.

The medication had no effect whatsoever, so I continued my downhill trajectory for a few months more. Sometime around

Easter of the next year, I went into hospital for surgery to bypass my duodenum, done by making a new hole in my stomach and attaching my small bowel to that, to allow me to eat some food.

This was when they told me I had Crohn's disease, that there was no cure, maybe it was genetic, but they could manage it for me. No mention of adverse reactions to any vaccine or anything, so still no link in my mind, or anyone else's. I remember two distinct things when getting this news. On the one hand, there was a deep sinking feeling. On the other, the relief that they knew what was wrong with me and were able to keep on top of things now. A good example of the instincts telling you one thing, your intellect telling you the opposite, and experiencing both at the same time.

Luckily, my school education in avoiding bullies by projecting a false persona proved very useful, allowing me to push away that sinking instinctual feeling, to go instead with the positive intellectual news, and pretend everything was good.

So there you have a little slice of my life, and I'm going to treat that moment of diagnosis as the starting point for my illustration of how solutions can maintain and exacerbate the original problem over a long time.

Maybe I could take it back further and start from the point of the vaccination. I say this because the BCG vaccine is to prevent TB (tuberculosis), and before Crohn's disease was called Crohn's disease, many knowledgeable people thought it was intestinal TB. But then they decided it wasn't when some bloke with a tongue-twister of a surname got it named after himself.

I could even go back further than the vaccination as the starting point. One very important thing regarding health is that many, many different influences must align before serious illness develops. So while I can state with some confidence that my Crohn's was triggered by a BCG vaccine, this is very different to saying the BCG vaccine causes Crohn's. Yes, it did for me, but this was only because my prior life had promoted the underlying conditions leading to such an outcome. For now, though, I'll go forward and explain a bit more about the path it set me on.

3

Following The Science

I'm going to be rather briefer regarding the events of the next 20 or so years. After my initial illness in 1986, followed by surgery and diagnosis in 1987, it took decades to start making any real sense of my predicament. I certainly don't want to use this book to moan about myself because doing such a thing isn't going to help with anything. However, I do need to give you a sense of just how bad my situation got, and how my perception of it gradually shifted over time, to add some context to the solution I have arrived at.

So, I was discharged from the hospital with a new exit inside my stomach, a great big scar running from top to bottom on the outside, and a prescription for some tablets that were going to keep my disease under control and make me feel well. The prescription was for prednisolone, a steroid used to treat inflammatory conditions.

The steroids worked marvelously. I soon felt more like my original self, fit and healthy, eating better, back to a decent weight, and life kind of returned to normal. All was well for the next couple of years, apart from an ongoing, nagging feeling that maybe it wasn't going to be quite that simple.

When I reached the age of sixteen, I was transferred to a hospital outpatient department for grown-ups, and the first thing they told me was that I had to stop taking prednisolone, because long-term usage is really bad for you. It's difficult to make a concise list of all the problems it leads to, but things like bone loss (in terms of losing calcium and other minerals out of them, not just losing bones in a 'where did I put that?' sort of way), heart troubles, stomach and intestinal ulceration(!), glaucoma, a big list of psychiatric problems, and the list goes on and on and on. So, I started on a slow reduction of my dose, the idea being that my body would adjust, everything would be fine, and I could then get on with normal life.

I should point out that back in the 1980s, pharmaceutical knowledge was the preserve of the medical industry. There was no internet to tell you about medicines and their associated problems. While there were physical libraries of actual books, the libraries near me didn't have anything along the lines of a medical reference section, the main focus of the stock being old, dog-eared romance or crime novels. Not that I would have done any research anyway, as both my trust and my perceived range of options were firmly rooted in the National Health Service.

Anyway, over a few months, I got my dose down to almost zero, but my general health also reduced in line with this. I began feeling more like I had when I first became ill three years earlier. Upon investigation, it was found that I had some new ulcers, this time around the new exit to my stomach, and these were affecting its revised drainage. I was very clever in being able to frame these as being a completely different form of ulceration to the Crohn's Disease in my duodenum, and as such didn't need to question the cause or potential solution.

Therefore, the doctors still held the keys to the repository of answers. The answer this time was omeprazole, at the time a new wonder drug, and this was because these new ulcers allegedly must have been due to overproduction of acid. I also had to go back on a high dose of prednisolone because the 'Crohn's' in my duodenum had taken the opportunity to 'flare' back up.

Strangely, my new issues were kind of a repeat of the first time around – diagnosis of ulcers, and therefore ulcer medication to treat them, and no discernible positive result. But definitely normal ulcers as opposed to Crohn's, and I believed it just the same as I believed the ulcer diagnosis the first time around. At least this time I suppose there was some sort of logical reason as to why someone so young might be developing ulcers, namely that there was a hole in my stomach where it wasn't designed to have one.

I'm writing this from the perspective of how I processed it all at the time. It was what the doctors were telling me, and nobody was telling me anything else, so that is what I went with. While they did tell me that long-term use of steroids could lead to ulcers, they didn't explain why. The answer, as far as I understand it now, lies at the bottom of a rather big can of worms, and I'll be addressing this once I've explained the trajectory of my life up to the present day. They also didn't tell me much about omeprazole, other than it would help heal the new ulcers, but it wouldn't have much impact on my Crohn's.

I now know, or at least strongly suspect, that in my case at least, the inflammation and ulcers defined as Crohn's exist for the same reasons as the ones not labelled as Crohn's, so to suggest that the same medicine can target one of them but not the other could arguably be seen as a bit of a sketchy claim.

Sketchy claims aside, omeprazole didn't help much. So I was instructed to take more of it. Taking more made me feel more unwell than I was to begin with, taking less of it or none didn't change much about how I felt, so over time I forgot to take it.

Returning to the side effects of prednisolone, the knowledge that one of these is gastric ulceration makes it seem somewhat bizarre to use such a thing to treat a disease that is, for all intents and purposes, gastric ulceration. And there we have the first snippet of what I set out to write about. Now, if I took it, and then got the associated problems straightaway, this would flag it up as something best avoided. But that isn't how things happened. When I was on a high dose, I felt good: I could eat food, and could generally get by fairly well. When I tried to reduce my dose, I'd suffer what is termed a 'flare-up', leading to the conclusion that I needed more prednisolone, and thus I developed an absolute dependence on it, ending up in a repeating cycle. Ultimately, it created a closed loop of facilitating the development of more of the disease it was being used to treat, thus necessitating more of it to keep everything under control, which then created more disease once again, and round and round it went. At the time though, I perceived this situation as a simple need to keep taking it, to keep my ill health at bay and stay well.

By this point I was aged seventeen, so had been the proud owner of my disease for about four years. I had still not made any link to the thing that kick-started the whole nightmare, namely my BCG vaccine. While I can trace my issues further back, it was the major trigger point for my physical deterioration, so I think I am justified in classing it as a major determining factor in how my illness came about. Please remember I'm not presenting a case for or against vaccines here. While I do have my own opinions regarding them, a wider discussion is not entirely relevant in terms of what I am writing about. The only thing I will say, and the medical industry agrees with me on this, is that a certain number of people are going to react particularly badly to any given vaccination.

One thing before getting back to my main narrative, and this is regarding areas that I'd argue are somewhat lacking from my history of medical care. First of all, I've never, and I mean not once, had any sort of allergy or intolerance testing done, other than a gluten intolerance test in 2022, some thirty-six years after first becoming ill. Looking back, maybe it would have been a good idea at some point, such as at the very start, to run some simple tests and see if I was reacting to one or more specific constituents of foodstuffs. But no. Second, maybe a detailed dietary analysis might have shed some light on my predicament. Again, no. I did have some interactions with dietitians, but the focus was on getting calories into me as opposed to whether anything specific was causing problems. I do remember being told many times that food was not the cause of Crohn's so I could eat whatever I wanted. The rather late-in-the-day gluten test I finally had came back negative, by the way. I had already been avoiding gluten for over a month when I finally got tested though, and it will only return a positive result if gluten is present in your system.

Anyway, back to where I was. The next few years were endless fun for me. Frequent trips to the hospital for emergency stabilisation, high doses of prednisolone for a while, then a gradually reducing dose until my next trip to the hospital for some more emergency treatment. I began to have ongoing problems with anaemia, which was attributed to malabsorption of iron or maybe ongoing bleeding, so I was prescribed iron tablets. These kept my haemoglobin level up for varying amounts of time until it invariably plummeted back down through the floor, sending me back to the hospital for repeated blood transfusions and ever higher doses of steroids.

My ability to eat enough to hold my weight was by this time entirely dependent on my medication, but as with all medicines, this ended up being a cycle of diminishing returns, meaning I was very often desperately underweight.

Words can't quite convey how difficult life is when you have something like this. I can state with absolute certainty that when you look as if you have just been rescued from a concentration camp, people mostly do anything they can to avoid you, so along with your ongoing lack of energy, you also get to experience some great discrimination. You do get some sympathy when you first become unwell, but after a while, that kind of dissipates. I don't want to assign any blame here, as I completely understand that it drains people to be around someone who is ill.

I wrote a whole load more about my experiences of being left out, passed over, and forgotten about, but when I read it back it just seemed like I was just indulging in my misfortune, so I deleted it. The only reason I'm mentioning this is because I do see an ever-increasing number of people whingeing and whining about how they have been downtrodden and discriminated against, and often wonder if they understand just how bad things actually can be. It is possible to argue that anyone who is really suffering, due to whatever reason, is going to be in the midst of such a struggle that they are not going to be in a position to tell many other people about it, so if you are hearing from somebody about their troubles, then maybe those troubles aren't quite as bad as they are being made out to be, or could be.

Back to my medication, I was next prescribed some

chemotherapy, via an immunosuppressant called azathioprine, as a way of ending my dependence on prednisolone, but that didn't work out very well. I ended up feeling even worse, so I went back to even more prednisolone. Azathioprine suppresses bone marrow, something that I've never felt too comfortable with anyway, so I wasn't too upset when it didn't help.

Aside from whatever treatments were prescribed, I did get plenty of well-meaning advice, where people advised me that I should eat more.

To this day, no amount of explaining seems to get through to some people, who just eat what they want when they want, have somewhere to put it inside of them, and don't then have to spend the next day, or several days, withstanding crippling pain while the food they ate tries to push its way through blockages. If you have never had such problems, you simply cannot appreciate them. More often than not, much of the food I ate would come back up at some point after having caused a whole lot of pain, so it was fairly pointless at best for me to take the advice and just eat more.

As I mentioned at the very start of this book, Crohn's Disease, for some reason I just can't fathom, just isn't up there with more headline-grabbing diseases, so isn't particularly well understood, which means people just don't always get how bad it can be. As well as making life even harder on a personal level, this picture also extends right up to the state level, and the welfare benefits that are available for ill and disabled people. In general, if you've got Crohn's, then you're getting nowt off the government while at the same time you're going to struggle with job opportunities, and with actually managing the requirements of a job, should you get one. This means you can be left in a very tight spot financially, something that provides a lovely bit of icing to go on top of the cake(*).

If you are in some sort of similar situation (in the UK, at least) and you feel that you need some help from the state, then my advice is to play the mental health angle when you make your claim. You will get much further if you can convince the authorities that you have severe anxiety as a result of your illness, rather than simply relying on the fact that you have an illness that makes you too ill to work. Being too ill to work is not seen as a good enough reason for anyone to opt out of work in the UK, whereas over-worrying is. I never got anything, but when I did try, I found the focus of the eligibility interview to be firmly centred on my mental rather than physical condition, and I wasn't prepared for that.

I could keep ranting on about this plenty more, but I started with the intention of passing on something useful. If you don't have this type of illness yourself then there is nothing I can do to convey how awful it is, other than suggesting you try to imagine what it would be like if you had a case of severe food poisoning, the kind where a few days into it you begin wishing you could just die. Then imagine this never coming to an end. If you do have some form of inflammatory bowel disease, then you might be recognising some of what I am saying. If so, my thoughts are with you – all I can say is hang on in there for the time being, and maybe something of what I've got to say might offer you some sort of path out of it, but please take the time to understand what I am saying, and don't just stop taking whatever medication you might already be on. The time to stop taking a medicine is when you don't need it any more, not when you just don't want to take it any more.

Something I can't stress enough is that even though one of

the themes of this book is about how pharmaceutical medicine is not the answer, there are times and situations where it might be the only thing keeping you alive.

Before returning to my actual story, I'll just provide a few extra breadcrumbs to anyone interested in psychological processes. I can't get to the bottom of this because I only know what I feel like, but it sometimes appears that other people respond differently to me in terms of the mental processes and coping mechanisms that come with an incurable illness. From my point of view, I've never felt as if I had Crohn's. This statement is difficult to qualify because I don't know how such a thing should feel. Even though I understand what I am told regarding my diagnosis, accept this is accurate, and even agree that pictures from scans and other tests make it clear that I have had a severe disease defined as Crohn's, I still never once felt like someone with such a thing. I can't be certain if anyone else ever does, but my observation is that some people seem to take to it much more readily than I have ever done.

What I mean by this is that sometimes people come across as if they feel like they have the disease that they have, as well as having its physical effects. I'm not a psychologist so can't really offer much more to what I am saying here, other than adding it could maybe be construed as some form of denial on my part, but there again I have always understood and accepted everything I have been told regarding the state of my digestive system. It's just that there's always been another part of me holding onto the idea that maybe I've not been seeing the full picture, and as such there has always been a path out of it if I could just find the route to take.

Back to the story of my life of illness, another treatment option that came about in the 1990s was the Elemental Diet

– complete nutrition in a liquid and mostly predigested form. It tastes awful, and treatment with it requires that you eat nothing else at all, and drink nothing else except water, which you don't want to do anyway since you are drinking Elemental drinks all day. I tried it a few times with some amount of success, at least over the very short periods of treatment. I've got a whole lot to write about the Elemental Diet but would be getting ahead of myself if I went into that now – trust me, though, I will be getting back to it, and it isn't good.

After a few long years of torment, I ended up back with the surgeons for a rework. They opened up what turned out to be numerous strictures in my small bowel, as well as recreating the secondary exit to my stomach, and this brought me back to life. A couple of years later I was back again, for more of the same, along with the removal of quite a bit of my small bowel, which was ulcerated beyond repair. While it is obvious that such a procedure removes a part of your physical self, something I can't quite explain is that along with this you lose some portion of your sense of self along with it. If you have ever seen the film *Johnny Mnemonic*, it explores such concepts, albeit for very different reasons. I can't tell you what I lost, because it isn't there anymore, but I know some part of myself disappeared with every bit of bowel that was taken out.

I don't know how much was removed. My surgeon was about to tell me once but I stopped him when he mentioned short bowel syndrome, as I felt that having this knowledge would have led to my mind solidifying much more in the way of restrictive behaviour and future expectations.

To help prevent yet more trips to surgery for more of the same, I started taking a daily dose of omeprazole once again, along with occasional courses of prednisolone, and some short-lived attempts to take another immunosuppressant, 6MP this time. 6MP is similar to azathioprine but it didn't make me feel quite so bad quite so quickly. However, it did make me feel just as bad after a time, so I would take it for a while, give up on it, and then try it again at a later date. This was the late 1990s. The doctors would no longer prescribe prednisolone as a long-term treatment because they said it was too bad in terms of side effects, and I'm not going to argue with that. So, how did omeprazole work out for me this time?

It seemed to help enormously this time, at least to start with. I got myself kind of on a stable footing for a few years. My symptoms seemed, for the most part, a bit more manageable. Since omeprazole isn't considered to carry the same risks as things like steroids and immunosuppressants, I took it every day and didn't worry too much about it. In my mind, it was holding the disease back, and keeping me away from the surgeons.

Up to this point my problems had all been in the upper parts of my digestive system. People with Crohn's tend to suffer from ongoing diarrhoea, but I had never had any such problems. My form of it had been exclusively in my stomach and small bowel. Earlier on in the trajectory of my disease, I would vomit every day or so. Not much of what I was eating was getting anywhere further than my stomach during those times, and I do remember occasionally thinking that the standard version of Crohn's, centred around diarrhoea, might have been a preferable option to my spewing-up version. Luckily for me, or rather, unluckily, I was about to discover why this wasn't the case at all.

Let's fast forward a few years now, by which time I was suffering regular and increasingly uncontrollable diarrhoea, something that developed very gradually. It turned out I now had Crohn's in my colon. Strange to say the least, since this had never once been a problem. Having had my disease for close to twenty years by the point I'm up to now, it seemed odd that it would just jump to a completely different part of my body and begin causing a whole set of new problems. It could be that the opening up of my upper digestive system, along with the removal of various pieces of it could have allowed whatever was causing my disease to get further through my system and thus start affecting lower parts of it. Thinking about this leads to the conclusion that the root cause is very definitely related to the content passing through the digestive system, and this is when I started to give such a notion much more attention. The doctors didn't agree though.

"Disease progression," they said, which is a very good explanation method for the medical industry. One of the industry's major selling points is the claim that it can prevent such things, yet they still get to play the disease progression card without any hint of contradiction. The medical establishment will quickly leap to the conclusion that a disease is just too aggressive to hold back, thus implying that the patient is the source of the problem. As a patient you never really hear concepts such as the treatment path, your diet, or both, adding massively to the underlying problem.

I'd argue that the medical perspective on nutrition is fairly basic and rudimentary, something that may seem like a bit of a bold claim. After all, people claiming to have a mastery of health should also be masters regarding the food we eat, but for many doctors and nutritionists, it is just stuff that we fuel our bodies with. The overall view is that as long as we follow the advice of some antiquated food pyramid with specific percentages of fat, protein, carbohydrate, and fibre, then there is nothing more food can offer in terms of health. You just have to look at the quality of hospital food to know that it is not ranked very highly on any scale of things required to promote health. People go into hospital for major surgery, or other medical emergencies, and are then given plates of slop to eat when they need to heal themselves.

I was beginning to make something of a link between the BCG vaccine and my Crohn's, but unfortunately didn't yet make any further links between my medication and new inflammation popping up in different places. So, following the advice of the doctors, I doubled down on my medicines and got much worse much more quickly.

"You have a particularly aggressive form of disease, we didn't get on top of it in time," was the explanation, along with, "We need to get even more aggressive with the treatment to get this under control."

So I tripled down on my medication, and got even worse again, even more quickly.

If you think you know about how bad diarrhoea can be, then in a small way, yes you probably do. It is something we all get to experience from time to time. If you have ever been forced to employ the tactics of an addict when purchasing toilet rolls, then you might also have an idea of how bad mine was.

It got to a point of being so bad that I was buying multipacks of toilet rolls every single day. I would go to different shops to fulfil my requirements, in much the same way that an alcoholic might spread their purchasing of cider around, or whatever else their alcohol of choice happens to be. I did the same thing for my bog roll, so I might have gone to Tesco or Morrisons one day, then

Home Bargains the next, B&M Bargains the day after, followed by the Co-op, or maybe the local Spar. This way I wouldn't get noticed too much by the staff in each shop. I'm not sure what difference it would have made in the grand scheme of things if the staff in a certain shop noticed I was buying way more of it than should have been necessary, but it did deflect some potential for embarrassment. I suppose I should be grateful it was still 2010 when this was happening, and not during the great toilet roll run at the start of the 'pandemic' of 2020.

I was still working full-time during all of this. To be able to go to work, I'd start the day with some diarrhoea, followed by some more diarrhoea, and then some more just before leaving for work. It was a twenty-minute drive to where I worked, which, fortunately for me was in a cinema in a large shopping centre, meaning there were lots of toilets. I had to leave home early every day, and this is because I would park as close as I could to the toilets nearest to the car park, run to those toilets for some diarrhoea, then walk through the shopping centre to the cinema, stopping off at toilets on the way for more diarrhoea. So the trip to work often took more than an hour. Luckily for me, I worked in the projection room, so I didn't have the added difficulty of being in front of customers. As long as the right films played in the right auditoriums at the right times, I was left relatively alone. So I could fit multiple diarrhoea breaks into my work day, obviously using different toilets where available, and going out into the shopping centre when possible to use the toilets there. At the end of a shift, I would do the reverse of my coming-into-work strategy. Once home I'd spend the rest of the day running up to the toilet very frequently and would then have a very broken night's sleep, due to having to get up at least once an hour for yet more diarrhoea. Then I would get up the next day, absolutely exhausted, and do the same all over again, remembering to keep a mental note of where I should buy my toilet roll from that day.

It took a while for things to get as bad as I have just described, but once it was that bad, it just went on and on for months, constantly getting a bit worse with each passing week. No amount of medication did anything to improve this. The word 'exhausting' doesn't get close to describing how hard it was to keep going. This state of affairs couldn't go on indefinitely.

By 2010, things had become so bad that I was sent back to the surgeons for the joy of getting a colostomy. I still have it to this day, I am stuck with it, I hate it, and will never get used to it, but I've learned to put up with it to an extent. I don't want counselling to come to terms with it. The only way I see of becoming happy with it is to learn to pretend I'm happy with it, and I've already spent too much time pretending. So I prefer to remain unhappy with it and just accept I am stuck with it. Up to a few years ago, I needed regular revisions of it, but even without repeated surgery, I am now tied to the medical industry forever more.

Just to put this into context, I don't mope around all day every day feeling sorry for myself (although people who know me might think differently on this matter). But in my mind, I don't. However, I reserve the right to not be happy with my stoma and all the associated difficulties that come along with it.

After this surgical intervention, I started to question the whole premise of pharmaceutical medicine. I had no idea as to what I might be able to do in place of it, so kept dipping my toes in and out of the water for several years to come. I was effectively convinced that I couldn't survive without omeprazole, and given my circumstances there was probably some truth in that concerning my immediate situation, so I continued taking it every day. However, I was beginning to seriously doubt the steroids, the immunosuppressants, and the new class of wonder drugs called monoclonal antibodies, also known as biologic drugs.

I stopped taking or refused to take all of those but let the doctors believe I was still taking them. This is because I thought they might withdraw all treatment if I refused to follow their prescriptions (which they couldn't, but I didn't know that). I would go back to anti-inflammatory treatments for periods when my resolve, or my health, weakened. My course of action, unfortunately, gave the doctors ammunition for their stance on the subject, as once they cottoned on to my scam of pretending to take their medicines, they were able to claim that the ever-worsening state of my colon was entirely due to my refusal to follow their advice diligently. They were never too keen to talk about why it had degenerated so badly in the first place when I had followed absolutely everything they suggested.

A strange occurrence was that my original, upper digestive disease seemed to settle down somewhat, correlating quite well with my self-directed reduction in constant anti-inflammatory medication. But now the doctors had engaged in a battle over my colon, so, from my perspective of how they were approaching it, they didn't notice the complete shift in symptoms. To them, it was the same disease, which required the same solution. I don't remember much ever being mentioned about why it was suddenly in a different part of my body and not where it had originally been. I do remember a great deal being mentioned about how my only chance of controlling it was to keep doing the very same things that hadn't managed to control it at all previously.

I got what is known as a loop colostomy to begin with, the idea being it might give my bowel a chance to rest, with the option to close it back up again. Then my bowel prolapsed out of it, and it is not entirely a fun experience when your insides fall out of a hole in your stomach. So I went back for a rework. Then the same thing happened again, so another revision of it followed. Then it retracted and closed up due to my skin growing over it, so needed further revisions each time this happened. I got it changed to an end colostomy, where it was detached completely from the remainder of my bowel, but it narrowed down and closed over again. So I got more revisions, including the removal of the end of my bowel, since having that left in but not functioning was deemed a high cancer risk. Every revision took a bit more of my colon away. Meaning I'm stuck with a colostomy forever now. All in all, I had about ten trips to surgery in as many years. I guarantee you that this takes its toll.

In terms of my timeline, I'm up to 2019 now, so 33 years from the initial onset of my disease (there's a good number for all you numerology-focused conspiracy theorists out there). It took a long time for me to begin falling out with the medical system, and once I did begin to change my perspective, it was a very slow and tortuous process. Up until I got my colostomy, sometime in or around 2010, I honestly hadn't questioned the medical approach too much. Once I did start to question it, I found myself in a very lonely and frightening place. I was beginning to realise that the medicines and surgeries were slowly killing me, but with the full knowledge that these were the only things keeping me alive on a day-to-day basis. This is the kind of situation that the word 'dilemma' was invented for.

Essentially, the choice I was seeing in front of me was either to continue with the treatments and cling on to whatever remainder of life such a path offered, or find a way to turn things around, but with the more immediate risk of not being able to survive at all.

Something that isn't talked about in medical circles, at least to patients, is the cumulative effect of repeated trips to surgery. The body doesn't have time to heal itself properly after each operation, and I'd argue particularly so if it is your digestive system, where the damage mounts up and up, resulting in increasingly aggressive inflammation. The medical doctors insist on throwing more and more drugs at the situation, way beyond any tipping point, where the medications only add to the damage without even providing any symptomatic relief. But they have no other options because all they can suggest are products from the pharmaceutical industry or yet more surgery.

In keeping with my lifelong strategy of avoidance, I had half-heartedly followed some of the medical treatments offered since getting my colostomy but then gave up on them when I thought better of it. There wasn't much of a choice to decline surgery after my original stoma prolapse scenario, as it then decided to keep closing up about a year after each revision, and the only option was emergency surgery to get it opened again. Other than this I just generally hoped that I would become better, or that my disease would somehow go away.

Throughout all of this, right from its beginnings way back in the 1980s, the dilemma I have just mentioned has always been there. Early on, I had always gone with the safe choice, the one where I would defer to other people claiming more knowledge and better qualifications than me about the best course of action for my ongoing state of health. Even as my health went from bad to worse, I generally stuck with what I perceived to be the safe option. My gradual refusal of treatment, which took about ten years to fully realise, was a pendulum starting to swing, but I didn't have much idea of where to take things from there. Because of this, I kept slipping back after taking steps away.

If you have never been in such a position, it can be very easy to say that you would accept the challenge to take charge of your situation and take responsibility for the outcomes of your self-directed actions. But would you do that? Really?

Let's not forget we are talking about life and death here. Medical intervention provides the option to continue being alive in the immediate term, whereas not accepting it brings with it the danger of a very rapid demise, particularly if you don't know what to do instead. We'd all like to think we have the resolve, and the nerve to forge our path through whatever lies ahead, but when there's already a seemingly nice and safe, well-lit road laid out in front of you, are you going to pass that up in favour of hacking your way through a pitch-black jungle?

Let's also not forget that once you have chosen the sensible option, and you are on that road of safety, you can very easily grow accustomed to it, and then you might have difficulty in terms of awareness of the ongoing sustainability of that road. If it becomes more narrow and less well-lit, such changes might be imperceptible if they occur over time.

In 1986 I took my first steps on the shiny and sparkly highway of medical disease management. By 2010 that had narrowed down to a single-track lane, full of twists and turns, with more than a few potholes, and without much in the way of lights to illuminate the way. By 2019 it was little more than an overgrown, unlit path. However, it remained more visible than whatever lay beyond the edges, and I had been on it for so long that I couldn't conceive of anything else.

It was going to take even more than I had been through up to this point for me to finally leave the path, the one that had once been that road of obvious choice.

In 2019 my situation finally started to push me into doing something about it.

4

It Doesn't Rain But It Pours

As I write this, my last trip to surgery was about four and a half years ago. My stoma had all but closed up once again, meaning it was causing a blockage right at the end of whatever digestive system I had left. This wasn't good, so the only option was to go back to the hospital and get it surgically revised.

I wasn't in too good a place in terms of general health when I went for this. My blood tests showed low levels of a variety of essential things, and this was because I hadn't been able to eat much for the several months my stoma had become a blockage rather than an opening. I was somewhat underweight as a result. In addition, the inflammatory markers in my blood indicated considerable active inflammation.

My surgeon wasn't expecting it to be too different from my previous few revisions, maybe a little more involved, but essentially just a tidy-up of my stoma, with perhaps an inch or two of my colon to be removed, then the new end of it would be stitched onto the opening in my stomach, meaning he felt I would be OK for surgery in the state of health I was in.

Once under anaesthetic and in the operating theatre, it was

found that a long section of my colon was badly inflamed and damaged beyond repair, so that was removed, and the remainder had to be stretched across my insides to reach the opening in my stomach wall. This was not good.

From the moment I woke up from surgery something felt very wrong, but I slowly began to believe the reassurances that it was all normal. It's strange how I can make myself believe such things, even with plenty of previous experience telling me otherwise. Anyway, I was then straight into the usual quandary presented to an in-patient at a British hospital. I needed to eat, but the hospital food was pretty much as bad as food can be, so I asked if I could go home to get some proper food and start recovering. After a few days I was discharged, so went home and then found I was unable to eat anything, and more worryingly I was also unable to drink anything. So I got back on the phone with the hospital intending to get re-admitted but only got to speak to a nurse, who decided I was simply constipated and therefore should take some laxatives (all of this over the phone, even though I was just 4 or 5 days out from surgery and was feeling genuinely terrible).

I managed to stay alive by sipping water for a few days, then upgraded to milk and slowly started to be able to eat small amounts. All of this at a time when my body was in desperate need of nutrients to heal up from surgery that had turned out rather more extensive than I was either physically or psychologically prepared for.

An appointment was already scheduled with my medical doctors (different from the surgical team) very soon after this, so I thought that would be my best chance to get someone to listen, and maybe start getting to the bottom of why I was feeling so bad. The appointment came, and as is becoming more common with medical appointments, the doctor performed a consultation with his computer screen while I sat there wondering why I had bothered to turn up, then he sent me for some blood tests before I went home.

Now then, I know when I am anaemic, and have so much experience of being anaemic that I know how badly anaemic I am at any time when I am anaemic. At this particular time, I guessed my haemoglobin level was somewhere around 70, which is a less-than-ideal place for it to be (it used to be measured on a scale going up to 14 but these days seems to be measured on a scale going up to 140). Using the modern scale, I don't feel any ill effects until it drops below 100. Once it is below 100, I begin to feel a bit unfit. Below 90 I start to get breathless more quickly than I should, even when doing basic things like going up the stairs. Below 80 the breathlessness expands to include light-headedness and occurs upon any exertion. Below 70 I start to feel particularly ill.

I told the doctor about it and that I was very concerned about it, so expected a call a day or two later to come in for an emergency iron infusion when my anaemia had flagged up on my blood tests. I also expected some kind of check for potential surgical complications. I heard nothing. I tried calling the hospital to get my results but got put on hold, then passed around, and got nowhere. So, I began to wonder if I was wrong and maybe just feeling a bit flat from the surgery and the rather bumpy recovery I was going through.

Three weeks later, a letter turned up at my door from the hospital. It told me my haemoglobin level was 70 and I should call my GP (General Practitioner) to arrange an iron infusion! Three weeks is a long, long time to endure with a Hb as low as that, especially when recovering from quite extensive surgery, and not being able to eat or drink properly at the same time. The intuitive part of me was thinking that I might have been bleeding internally.

So I called my GP who performed some blood tests and sent me off to another hospital the very same day as an emergency admission. My Hb was down to below 60 by now, which is getting into life-threatening territory. Another thing about having such low iron is that you cannot make any rational decisions, so while it might seem like the obvious choice to simply go to the emergency department, this kind of thought doesn't form. The other hospital gave me an immediate blood transfusion, and an iron infusion, followed by another a few days later.

I should have taken this up with my main hospital, as the way I see it, it ranks as one of those shocking moments where my perspective of the world changed for the worse, and someone should have been held accountable. However, I was entering into a whole world of new problems at the time, and as such never got around to raising a complaint.

Effectively, I felt abandoned by my regular doctors, who didn't seem to want to engage. This was in the year before the excuse of a pandemic would have been offered as a reason, so the NHS was, at that point, allegedly still running the same as it had been previously, with the word 'badly' being the best description I can think of for it.

The British health service is one of those things that British people believe is the best in the world, and this is because that is what we get told from a very early age. I'm not sure if this is still a thing, but on top of that, when I was young we were also told our army was the best in the world. I remember feeling genuinely sorry for people in other countries since I was lucky enough to live in the country with the best healthcare available, and the best fighting force ever to have existed. I never realised that every developed country tells its children the very same thing, and as such wondered what it must be like to grow up somewhere where they had to tell the next generation that another country was so much better than them in every respect.

So, back to me, I got to see a bunch of different doctors for the new problems that came up. As well as issues flagged up by my blood, my skin began disintegrating around my revised stoma and turned into nasty open sores, something I have never experienced before, and something I never wish to experience again. These were an instance of pyoderma gangrenosum (go look that one up for some lovely bedtime browsing if you have the stomach for it). I only found out what it was at a much later date – I at least had the sense, at the time, to take some photos of it. At the time though, I had the problem of not being able to get to talk to the surgeons, even though the surgeons tell patients to get back in touch if they have any problems. The way the NHS works is that the top people (i.e. surgeons and the like) are shielded from their patients by layers of bureaucracy. The pathway to them requires going through people at lower grades who will raise your case up the ladder when they think it is required. This is understandable in terms of maintaining a functioning system, as the surgeons would end up spending all of their time fielding silly questions and stupid concerns from people who don't have anything to worry about, but it means you are going to struggle when you do need to speak to someone, and you have to convince someone else who doesn't necessarily have the training or experience to decide that you need to see the specialist.

In life, you sometimes think you know about how painful

pain can be, and I've got plenty of experience of it to draw upon for such knowing. Regarding my skin situation, I'd never experienced pain quite like it, so phoned every contact I had in the NHS, and nobody wanted to help. This got so bad I even took myself to the casualty department at one point and was promptly sent back home with some bandages and sticky plasters, so that turned out to be a bit of a pointless exercise. Feeling as if there was nowhere to turn, I struggled on as best I could. Eventually, the sores began to settle down. I still have the indents on the surface of my stomach where it had been eaten away, or maybe more accurately, had disintegrated.

So that came and went, my anaemia seemed to stabilise, and the other markers in my blood that had been somewhat haywire also slowly returned to something resembling normal, and I went back to work, still feeling rotten, suffering a lot of discomfort and pain in my stomach, and still struggling to eat anything like enough food. After a couple of months, and on one particularly long shift at work (driving and delivering fruit and veg at this time – a computer had replaced me at the cinema several years before this), I started to get some rather worse pains and then began to vomit blood.

In true working-class fashion, and because I was quite a distance from home, I decided I would finish my shift, and then drive directly to a hospital that knew my medical background. I know that this will sound ridiculous when reading it, but when you are in an actual situation like this, common sense goes out of the window. Add into the mix the fact that I have either lost or have come very close to losing, every single job I have ever had because of my health.

When you are ill, yet still have to work, you are loath to not fulfil your duties, for fear of not being able to keep your only form of employment and therefore money to survive. You might ask why I was at work at all, and this is a question I have asked many times. As I mentioned earlier, I have even asked the system this very thing, in the form of applying for disability benefits. However, being half starved to death and physically unable to eat food just doesn't seem to tick the required boxes, and the system has always said no whenever I've asked for help, so I have been forced to go out and find work to pay my way. I wouldn't have it any other way now, because I prefer to take as little as possible from the government, but there have been times when I needed their help and got nothing. My general understanding of this is that there is a welfare state to help people in need, but if your name is Kevin Kendall then you can just piss off and sort yourself out.

Anyway, I got to the third last of nearly 100 deliveries over a 150-mile route, was just about home and dry, and was close to being able to drive to the casualty department back in Newcastle to have my life saved.

Then I vomited some more blood. A lot more. I was parked down a deserted back lane in a quiet part of a small town out in the middle of nowhere. I promptly blacked out, then came to, and spewed some more blood. I also started bleeding out of my stoma, quite significantly. I was feeling very weak and cold, and looking at what was coming out of me decided I had to call for an ambulance there and then. As I was out in the middle of the wilds of Northumberland, it took half an hour for an ambulance to get to me, and over that half hour, I began to feel what I can best describe as my lights going out. It was getting dark, the lane I was in led to nowhere, there was nobody there, and it was unlikely anyone would happen to pass by. Not that anyone passing by could have done much, but I've never felt so alone as I did for that half hour. I devoted all the will I could find to staying awake, and after what seemed like a lot longer, the blue lights of the ambulance finally made their appearance.

I was taken to yet another hospital, and can't quite remember what happened there, but ended up alive. I do remember them performing an emergency endoscopy where they found a large gastric ulcer that had been the source of at least some of my bleeding. All just three months after surgery that removed all of the diseased parts of my bowel. Since it was a different hospital, it was a different team of medics who provided this treatment, and they didn't know the full extent of my history. They brought me back to life, and I am eternally grateful for this, but they weren't in a position to tie in what was going on to the few months I had just experienced.

So, the endpoint of this long story is that when I finally went back to my gastric specialists, they also didn't tie together all the things that had happened, because, in the space of three months, I'd had a variety of treatments from several different hospitals.

I told my regular specialist doctors that I was convinced something had gone very wrong with the recent surgery, but my regular doctors were not the surgeons, and they were concerned specifically with my underlying inflammatory disease. They sent me for a CT scan to placate me, and it showed high levels of inflammation.

"Crohn's Disease,' they said, 'you need medication."

I'm not disputing the fact that inflammation was present. However, given the few months I had just endured, I thought surely they were going to look into what was causing this, and maybe come up with a decent course of action to resolve such high levels of a disease that should have been off the radar for some years, since the disease that had been there had just been hacked out and thrown in a bin somewhere, or maybe sent to a lab somewhere for some researchers to chop it up and do some dodgy experiments with. There again, given the quality of hospital food, I wouldn't be entirely surprised if it had found its way into that evening's nutritious and tasty meal.

However, it was plain and simple, "It's Crohn's disease, so you need monoclonal antibodies."

I refused.

"Well, you need some Chemo drugs to suppress your bone marrow." Feeling somewhat lost and confused, I started on a course of 6MP, then thought better of it, so stopped taking it.

"You still have severe Crohn's. You do need monoclonal antibodies."

I refused again.

Take a look at how monoclonal antibodies are manufactured, and if you get past the fluff that makes them seem all good, I promise you will think twice before embarking on a course of them.

The production of them sometimes involves live animals such as mice, other times it is done in a test tube, but whatever way it is done it involves cancerous cells and inoculations to make those cancerous cells produce antibodies. There is even a marketplace within pharmaceutical circles where companies can buy genetically engineered mice designed to develop the best sort of tumours for this process. If it is the live mouse method then the antibody production also involves mushed-up mice, but whether it is the mouse or test tube method, it involves mushed-up cancer cells. Obviously, these are all removed by some magical process and the resulting 'medicine' is 100% pure, uncontaminated antibody. Even notwithstanding the fate of the mice, it seems to me that making medicines this way is never going to lead to anything good.

However, the pharmaceutical industry is beyond reproach, so the monoclonal antibodies being injected into people are completely pure and entirely safe, meaning there's nothing to worry about.

By the way, I have a bridge to sell if you are interested.

Anyway, I had just come about as close to death as I ever have. While I had been slowly climbing over the fence regarding the mainstream medical approach to Crohn's for several years, I still had no real alternative. I would like to be able to say my near-death experience gave me the push I needed to change my situation, but I have a sneaking suspicion that without the events that were about to play out, I would still be stuck in much the same predicament to this day, or more probably an even worse one.

In late 2019, just when I was struggling in a very real way to cling to my life, stories started appearing in the media about a new, highly contagious, and deadly disease emerging out of Wuhan, China. And so began the story of Covid-19.

This came about at what could be seen as just about the worst possible time for me. I was in no position to be able to withstand a killer flu on top of all my other ongoing and worsening problems. As with everything in life, though, there are always different ways to perceive and approach things.

I didn't know how to deal with my Crohn's, but was by this point fully aware that the accepted medical path was no help whatsoever. One effect of acquiring this knowledge was that I began to wonder about a great many other things. If all the specialists and professionals in the field of Crohn's could be wrong in how they understand it and treat it, then what else could medical science, or just science in general, be getting, or have gotten wrong?

Rather than adopting a fear-based strategy and preparing for the alleged upcoming pandemic by hiding and trying to protect myself, I decided, once and for all, to take the bull by the horns. The perceived threat of Covid was the defining moment for me to find a way to stop taking all of my medication, and to make myself healthy enough to survive whatever this new flu turned out to be.

Initially, I didn't get off to a great start. For one thing, I couldn't resolve my need for omeprazole. Then I came down with a cold or maybe the flu over Christmas 2019 and was flattened by it. Not Covid-19 apparently, because it hadn't made it to these shores by then. Just some other cold or flu-type thing, with every single one of the symptoms that were soon to be associated with Covid, but no, it couldn't possibly have been actual Covid.

Some blood tests that had been taken just before this had flagged severely low levels of Vitamin D, so my doctors prescribed a very high dose of it. Now, given the stance of doctors when it comes to vitamins, my levels must have been really low for them to prescribe it to me. Typically it isn't something they do, even though I've had decades of malnutrition to contend with.

I started feeling a bit better as a result, and this had the effect of joining a few dots in my mind. Not just better from the not-Covid symptoms I'd spent more than a week suffering from, but a general feeling of calm and well-being that had been very lacking since the trip to surgery I have just told you that long story about. The dots that joined up were related to nutrients, and how I needed to get more of them into me. I have tried to come up with another way of describing this, as it seems like a bit of a statement of the obvious, but the joining up of the dots did just bring about the simple realisation that the way to heal myself was to get as many nutrients into my body as I possibly could.

A bit of research led me to the conclusion that the prevalence of cold and flu is linked to levels of vitamin D, and also vitamin C. I have found nothing in medical literature to extend this link to a lack of these being potential causative factors, but my reasoning led me to think that if I did whatever I could do for myself to improve my relevant vitamin levels, then I could only place myself into a better situation should I get a respiratory virus. And since I hadn't had Covid, evidenced by the fact that the government wasn't ready with its response by then, I had no desire to catch an even worse cold than the one I'd just had.

A big step on my route out of having to keep my disease was a high dose of vitamin D3, along with an even higher dose of vitamin C.

If you decide to take either of these, high-dose vitamin D3 might be better taken in combination with vitamin K2, as this is claimed to prevent the risk of arterial calcification, something that is said to be a possibility. Vitamin C might be more appropriate in its buffered form, spread into small amounts across the whole day, so Sodium Ascorbate as opposed to Ascorbic Acid. This prevents indigestion for one thing but also removes the danger of the acid leaching minerals out of your body to buffer itself once inside of you.

As with everything I'm discussing here, I'm not an expert, so cannot provide you with risk profiles of taking such things at high doses, and can't tell you whether they will be good for you or not. If you embark on any course of action for yourself, then you need to do the relevant research into what you intend to do and accept the potential risks.

Anyway, 2020 got underway, and the media joined with the government and a certain global health organisation, to gradually whip up stories and fears about the dangers of the ensuing pandemic. At the same time, I managed to start making some inroads into my own health crisis. I also started to realise that a person's actual underlying state of health is by far the most important factor concerning the development of an illness and that whether or not that disease is spread via a contagion is of much less importance. This helped me stop worrying about Covid-19, as I was able to focus on goals that would, in principle, lessen the impact of whatever it turned out to be.

5

The Sky Is Falling Down

Fear is a strange thing. It can affect the decisions you make to such an extent that those decisions are arguably no longer your own. When you are in the grip of fear, you will readily defer to anyone or anything offering a route out of that state.

Generally speaking, if you have something wrong with you, then doctors and medicine are there to step in. Whether this helps with your illness or not is only part of the story though. The other thing on offer is a mitigation of the fear that comes with being unwell. There's no better way of doing this than consulting with an expert who knows all the ins and outs related to whatever is wrong.

In early 2020 I found myself in a situation where the medical industry had done nothing to help alleviate my fears, having instead done quite the opposite. The issues surrounding my surgery in 2019 had a lot to do with this, including the horrendous aftercare provided by the NHS. In addition, the doctors insisted that I should just continue with the same treatments they had suggested many times before.

If you dig down into where fear comes from, and if you dig far enough, its roots are always tangled up with death. It is fairly easy to see this association when looking at health-related fears. Everything being offered by the health service was bringing my fear of death more into focus rather than dissipating it. So why am I telling you this now?

The answer is that I am about to tread on some rather delicate ground, and as such I need to be as clear as I can be about where my mind was when all of this happened.

I still wasn't feeling well at all and was convinced the treatments I had received over many years were now more of a problem than the original disease. Yes, I know much of that treatment had been of the life-saving variety at the times it was administered, but I was also starting to formulate some ideas that might have been much better if only they had been applied to my illness much earlier, such as from the start. I was also beginning to wonder why doctors were completely unreceptive to any alternatives.

Please don't confuse my use of the word 'alternative' here. I am talking about actual alternatives to the standard medical approach, but ones that have definite causes and effects. This is in contrast to many alternative health or healing options. I have a very analytical mind and need to be able to directly see actions and effects. Just like a scientist, in fact.

I have a considerable dislike of ambiguity, meaning if I can't see all of the steps to a process, I'm not interested in it. So, for me, this rules out most forms of what is commonly referred to as alternative therapy.

Concerning the medical system and my doctors, I got to see something I can only describe as institutional psychopathy, by which I mean an unwavering focus on increasing the toxic load on my body when my body couldn't withstand much more of it. Even when the doctors had a lifetime's worth of my medical notes demonstrating that none of the treatments had ever helped overall, they still insisted on going with them. I was starting to see recommendations of medicines as being nothing more than a sales pitch.

You might think of double glazing or used car salespeople as typical stereotypical examples of how the hard sell technique works. However, you may also want to add doctors to your list.

I'm paraphrasing here, but have been subjected to the following kind of exchange with doctors numerous times since giving up on the standard medical approach, and this started getting intense in 2020 when I was taking more determined steps to remove myself completely from prescribed medicine...

Doctor: *You have severe inflammation. You need monoclonal antibodies.*

Me: *I'm not doing that. I'm not convinced they are safe or effective.*

Doctor: *Of course they are. Studies prove it. They will give you a definite percentage of improvement in your condition.*

Me: *How many people suffer serious adverse reactions?*

Doctor: *Just a small number. You don't have to worry about that. You should worry more about your inflammation.*

Me: *Even if less than one percent of one percent of people react badly, each person in that tiny percentage is going to suffer one hundred percent of whatever adverse events occur.*

Doctor: *Yes, but that's a risk worth taking.*

Me: *Can you say whether I will be in the small percentage of adverse reactions or not?*

Doctor: *No, but that risk is insignificant compared to the risks of not managing your inflammation.*

Me: *But if that insignificant risk does happen to me, then I'm going to be in a much worse position than I am now.*

Doctor: *But it is your best option.*

Me: *I happen to think not. These 'rare' events include the likes of death, unusual cancers, serious infections, and liver or kidney failure. Aside from the immediate risks, what are the long-term effects?*

Doctor: *These are new, cutting-edge therapies. We don't envisage too many long-term problems.*

Me: *Well, you can envisage all you like. Another way of framing that would be to say you have no idea. Are there cases where people respond well to begin with, but then develop increasing intolerance to monoclonal antibodies?*

Doctor: *Yes, but we have other ones to prescribe if that happens.*

Me: *I don't think this is a good risk. If such a thing is something that happens, there must be something in these medicines that the body isn't too happy about. I'll pass on this treatment.*

Doctor: *In that case, you need some Chemo drugs to suppress your bone marrow.*

Me: *Are they safe?*

Doctor: *Mostly, yes. A small number of people develop problems.*

Me: *Will I be one of that small number?*

Doctor: *Nobody knows. It is worth the risk though. You have severe inflammation.*

Me: *But what if I am in that small number?*

Doctor: *The chances are you won't be.*

Me: *It mentions lymphomas in the side effects. Also liver or kidney failure, and increased infection risk. Similar risks as with the monoclonal antibodies.*

Doctor: *Yes, but we can monitor your blood in case problems arise.*

Me: *But if that happens and one of those things flag up in my blood then I'll also be on the way to having cancer or liver failure or kidney failure by the time it shows up.*

Doctor: *It wouldn't get to that point. Anyway, we have specialists in these areas if any problems do develop.*

Me: *I would say that if I ever need to see one of those specialists, then given my underlying condition, the only specialist help they* will be able to provide is in managing my path into an early grave.

Doctor: *But this is just a very small risk.*

Me: *But you won't know if it is going to cause one of those things until it has caused it, and I'm not overly confident with this kind of a scenario.*

Doctor: *You need treatment for your inflammation though.*

Me: *What is causing my inflammation?*

Doctor: *Nobody knows. But we can manage it. It might be genetic.*

Me: *I'm the only person in my entire extended family to have ever had anything like this, so the genetic theory doesn't stand up. I contend that since you don't know why I have this inflammation, you are not in any position to tell me how and why I should get rid of it. I don't want any of what you are offering.*

Doctor: *You need to take something. If you don't you will end up having your entire digestive system removed, and we will have to feed you through a tube in your vein from that point on. And you will get cancer and die because of that. I am the expert in these matters, so you are in no position to argue about these treatments.*

(More than one doctor has actually said that to me)

Me: *I'd rather take my chances with the entire digestive system removal or the unspecified cancer thing I'm apparently going to get if I opt to not take the drugs with potentially catastrophic consequences.*

Doctor: *You are putting yourself into an even more dangerous situation by not taking anything.*

Me: *But if I happen to be one of that small number of people who develop serious problems, then such an outcome would surely be the more dangerous one.*

Doctor: *But that is unlikely to happen.*

Me: *But what if it does?*

Doctor: *The potential benefit outweighs the potential risk.*

Me: *If they happen to affect me negatively, then you still get to weigh this against whatever positive results you see in other patients, in whatever time frame you make your measurements over. But to me, it will not matter how many positive results you have had if I get the negative ones.*

Doctor: *This is your best option, though*

Me: *I'm also not going to take my omeprazole anymore, by the way.*

Doctor: *(turns into Lemongrab from the cartoon Adventure Time)* UNACCEPTABLE!!!

I haven't seen a doctor turn into Lemongrab (if you have no idea what I'm talking about, go onto YouTube and search

"Lemongrab Unacceptable"), but I have been subjected to everything else in this example conversation, and it does give you the gist of the sales tactics of doctors. Essentially it comes down to them presenting your only options as either doing exactly what they say or dying a horrible death. It is hard to refuse under these terms, but since I was convinced that these treatments were now the main cause of my ongoing disease, I stood my ground.

Jumping forward a bit, I have successfully reduced my inflammation all by myself now, but I haven't quite reached that point in my story yet.

At the start of 2020, I was still taking omeprazole. It comes in capsules full of little granules. I decided to reduce my dose very slowly, so opened the capsule each day, removed some granules, and then took the remainder as normal. I removed a few more granules whenever I felt able to. It took more than a year to get my dose down to zero, during which time I realised that for me it had led to even more dependence than prednisolone, which itself is renowned for its properties of physical addiction.

Anyway, the point of me telling you all of this, apart from it being part of my ongoing narrative, is that I was in no way receptive to anything any medical expert was telling me at the time, so I had a lot of suspicions regarding everything I was hearing about an upcoming pandemic. I knew the experts were wrong regarding my health, and the experts on my health have all the same checks and balances as any other health expert to prove they cannot be wrong. Yet wrong they are.

I'm not going to discuss the Covid-19 story too much, even though I do have some very strong views on everything that has transpired due to it and is still transpiring.

For one thing, I don't want to get side-tracked from the main focus of this book, because what I have to say about Crohn's is too important. Also, I want this book to remain available and visible on major online platforms, and some of what I would like to say about Covid does not align with the current stance of those platforms.

What I will say is that after a little bit of initial acceptance of the story, I saw the same fear-inducing tactics that I'd been subjected to for my Crohn's, and as soon as I saw those I couldn't believe a single word coming from the mouth of anyone pushing the narrative of doom. This included government and public health officials, from the local level right up to the international, as well as the media. I had faced a whole lot of very real fear in the months leading up to the rollout of the propaganda surrounding Covid, so didn't respond by going into a panic. As such, I didn't enter into the correct state of mind to defer my decision-making to any alleged higher authorities.

Against this backdrop, my slow reduction of omeprazole was something of a rough experience. I got to feel all of the symptoms it had been masking, so suffered lots of really bad indigestion, probably a few minor bleeds in my stomach and small bowel, and a lot of difficulty eating anything. Out of all of the steps I took to end my dependence on pharmaceuticals, it felt as if getting free of omeprazole was the most risky.

In the middle of my own personal struggle, I was then expected to worry more about Covid than anything else in history. What I saw though, was more of the hard selling tactics I had been refusing to go along with for my predicament, the only real difference being that this new sales pitch was aimed at everyone instead of just ill people. At its most basic, this can be summed up as a demand to suspend the instincts and give all decision-making over to someone else.

When the lockdowns started, I was technically in an at-risk category due to my other health problems. I say this in terms of how Covid was being presented, not in terms of whatever the reality was. Given the previous year, I decided to rely on my instincts, which were telling me the real threat came from the people demanding my unquestioning acceptance.

I could very easily have shut myself in my house and stayed there for a very long time. Instead, I remained at work, and since my job was food delivery and thus a key worker position, this meant going out. I increased my hours and drove around empty streets delivering my fruit and veg, and have to say it was all somewhat surreal. In effect, the lockdowns worked in reverse for me.

I also refused to wear a mask, got bullied in shops for my noncompliance, didn't partake in the hand-sanitising thing, wasn't bothered about social distancing, didn't queue up for any PCR tests, and faked the lateral flow tests my employer insisted I do twice a week (although if I'm still working in my current job and someone higher up in the company happens to read this, then obviously, I'm just making all of this up). When not at work, I flouted the rules regarding only going out once a day, by walking the dog whenever possible, visiting family, and then finding ever more superfluous reasons to go to the shops for 'essential' supplies.

I didn't catch Covid once, other than the thing I had in late 2019 that was exactly the same, months before it was possible to be Covid, meaning it wasn't Covid that I had, but some other less dangerous illness, albeit with identical symptoms.

I was still struggling tremendously with my aim of stopping taking omeprazole though. While I was certain it was a major factor regarding the issues with my colon, I was in something of a vicious circle with it. So the dose I gave myself fluctuated. I'd reduce it when I felt I could, but then increase it when I thought I might be about to have a serious bleeding incident, or at times when my indigestion simply became too unbearable to put up with. This was made even more concerning by the effective closure of the health service, which was repurposed overnight into a Covid service, meaning I felt I was going to struggle even more if my self-directed drug reduction experiment led to any serious problems. As it turned out, though, I was in a category of such serious illness that I still got to go into hospitals and still saw doctors. The medical stance regarding my disease was that I was so ill with it that I still needed to be seen, even when the hospitals had closed their doors to almost everyone else. So I got to go into hospital a few times. As with my surreal experience of empty roads while at work, I also got to see the inside of empty hospitals.

One time I was sent for an MRI scan, which meant going to the main X-ray department. I went in, expecting to see Covid patients littering the corridors, because I still thought there must be something to the whole narrative, even if that something was very far removed from the proclamations of the government and their behavioural insights team. After all, a respiratory disease that induced severe breathing difficulties would surely mean X-ray would be stressed to breaking point. But it was empty.

Another time I had to go in for an iron infusion, probably because I'd pushed my omeprazole reduction too fast, resulting in more bleeding than I could deal with on my own. As with the MRI scan, I attended an almost empty hospital.

As well as my situation at the time, there is more to why I wasn't falling for the story. Much of my attention at that time was focused on how all the medical interventions I had received over the years had ended with me having to take major risks to get free of omeprazole, so I wasn't about to listen to a bunch of politicians or health officials. Added to this, my educational background tells me that public health officials have more in common with data analysts than they do with actual clinicians.

While I am not medically qualified, I am qualified in computing, and as such can state with confidence that data analysis can be heavily influenced due to bias, expectation, and sloppy coding. My background was in low-level programming, specifically with geometry pipelines for 3D graphics engines. I know better than most people, professors of public health included, about the limits of accuracy when working with fractional numbers inside a computer. Numbers with a decimal point have limits and blind spots, which are small enough to seem insignificant. However, when you run a series of several thousand calculations on a set of numbers, all of those little blind spots and rounding errors add up. In programming, this effect is known as drift. With graphics programming, since the result of the calculations is images on a screen, it is plainly obvious to such a programmer that drift is a serious problem if it is not addressed. Since I know about the representation of numbers inside computers, I can also state categorically that using double-precision numbers does not solve the problem of floating point drift. I'm not sure that all areas of academic research can say the same though. The upshot of such an effect is that a seemingly solid model for something can produce wildly inaccurate results, even for a flawless dataset and code implementation, even though such a scenario is simply not possible anyway. Add into this equation the fact that datasets can have a whole range of additional biases built in, and it soon becomes obvious that any computer model of future events can very easily produce utter garbage. A great deal of bias comes from the fact that any model of the real world must set boundaries in terms of the variables being manipulated, meaning assumptions must be applied. These assumptions can be no other than articles of faith and are likely to be very heavily influenced by the person writing the code, as well as by the requirements of whoever is providing the funding for the research - modern science does not operate within a vacuum.

Apologies for that long paragraph, but it is really important to make a very clear distinction between actual science and data modelling. Data modellers, sitting in their ivory towers behind their prestigious titles, are not scientists.

To illustrate this, let's say someone wanted to know what would happen if a pile of mud was prodded with a stick, a seemingly simple proposition.

A data modeller would define the stick and the pile of mud mathematically, create an algorithm to look at the potential interactions of these, run that algorithm many times to generate a set of potential outcomes, and then plot the results on a graph showing probable outcomes. From that, they would declare their discoveries and conclusions.

An actual scientist would find lots of sticks and make lots of piles of mud, and would then prod the different piles with different sticks to see what happened. A real person will, after much prodding, begin to gain an intuitive sense of what will happen in various situations, and will then be able to predict with some accuracy what might happen in different scenarios. This is something that most people have some sort of sense of, due to investigations carried out in early childhood with the aforementioned sticks and piles of mud.

A computer program is not capable of developing any intuition whatsoever, so it must encode every possibility into every calculation. This might seem fairly simple for something like sticks and mud. However, a stick has a great many properties. These include length, thickness, straightness, rigidity/elasticity, consistency of overall dimension, moisture content, saturation point of the fibres, knots and branches, decay level, prior or current infestation, effects of the conditions it was grown under, along with an endless range of irregularities in each factor throughout. Mud consists of sand, gravel, clay, and moisture, all in varying proportions and distributions, can contain any number of unknown contaminants, will have plant, fungal, and animal matter, both dead and alive within it, will contain worms, insects, or other creatures, or even just the results of those creatures' prior endeavours. The shape of the mud can be anything, and it might have gaps of various sizes in it, with varying distributions of moisture throughout. The surrounding environment will also affect the qualities of both the stick and the mud, and the prodding method will further affect any outcome – speed, force, distance, and direction, to name but a few factors. Due to the underlying complexity of the sticks and the mud, the only real way of developing any sort of accuracy would be to implement a particle system right down to the molecular level, something that is excessively intensive in terms of both computing resources and development time. I could probably come up with plenty more factors, but even with the ones I have mentioned, it is quite impossible to encode every possibility for each into a simulation, leading to a requirement for assumptions and drastic approximations. Because of this, the best any computer model can do is provide a very rough estimate of what might happen when the mud is prodded with the stick.

It should be obvious that if you look at the example of doing some actual prodding, it is impossible to prod every kind of mud with every kind of stick in existence. Hence the modern reliance on data modelling to find answers. However, data modelling suffers from even more of the same problem, in that the modellers must be able to define limitless variations in both the sticks and the piles of mud. They can't do such a thing, so they must then build a model within limits.

Unfortunately, the world is captivated by computers, so if a data modeller produces a set of results for their stick-prodding-mud model, it is assumed to be the definitive answer. At least if you are doing some actual prodding, you can specify the limits to your results, or if you claim too much from your investigations, other people can easily see those limits.

In the world of modelling, human nature will invariably lead to exaggerated claims regarding the robustness of any model. It is no simple matter to refute predictions, with or without the numerical drift I mentioned before. There are always flaws in algorithmic logic, along with the implementation of that logic. It requires a very high level of skill in computer programming to be able to find such flaws, along with a programmer who can be bothered to pick through the finer details of someone else's code, something that isn't enjoyable in any way whatsoever.

Hopefully, you will agree that even trying to model all the potential effects of prodding mud with a stick is quite impossible, beyond some very basic approximations within tight limits. Producing a model of how some brand new disease will impact the entire world is of an entirely different order of magnitude to models of sticks and mud, but in 2020 we all were being told these models were scientific fact. I honestly think that people in government and academia, for the most part, do believe they are dealing in facts with these kinds of things and this is because most of them are not computer programmers. This applies particularly to those in government, but also to a large proportion of academics and scientists who wrongly believe a computer is just another tool, in the same way a microscope is. As such, most cannot understand that the computer models are telling them nothing more, and nothing less, than what they want to be told.

As a programmer myself, I can state with absolute certainty that as a tool, a computer is more like a mirror than a magnifying glass. It tells you exactly what you tell it to tell you. I could go on and on, and then on some more, but I'm not writing this book to try and convince you about the intricacies of either Covid-19, whatever it is, or the nature of computers.

So ends the story of 2020 for me. The one positive thing it did was to fix my attention completely on managing my disease by myself. The only thing left to do was to find out what was causing it. Oh yes, and stop needing to take omeprazole.

6

Getting Elemental

Towards the end of 2020, I had some blood tests for inflammatory markers. Of note, if you know about such things, my CRP (C-reactive Protein) was somewhere around 30, and my faecal calprotectin was at something above 2500. If you know about these tests, then I'll confirm that yes, I have just given you the correct figures.

A year later, at the end of 2021, my CRP was at about 9, and my calprotectin was around 1000, so each was less than half the level it had been at a year earlier. This was over a year during which I had managed to come off all of my medication and had started looking very much more closely at treating myself with something that worked.

Now, once more, if you know anything about these tests, then yes, the 2021 figures are still very high, and would have indicated to any doctor that I was going through a full-on flare-up of my disease, hence the sales pitch for medication every time I spoke to them.

However, between these two times, I reduced the figures without any intervention from the pharmaceutical industry. So even though they may appear to have still been somewhat high in 2021, I had survived with them twice as high a year earlier. I've no idea what they might have been in 2019 when I had my disintegrating skin, followed by severe gastric bleed and near-death experience, but they were probably even higher again then.

During 2021 I finally managed to stop taking omeprazole altogether, but still didn't feel overly good in myself, understandably so if the above figures have any meaning for you. Without omeprazole, and without any immunosuppressants to mask my symptoms, I started to build up a better picture of what was causing problems in my digestive system. This was the first time in thirty-six years I had been completely medication-free. To start with, problems were due to any food I ate. At the start of a day, I wouldn't feel too bad, relatively speaking, but as the day progressed my indigestion and pain would increase directly in line with the quantity of food I had eaten. There was a delay of a few hours between eating and the onset of suffering, and it only went away after getting a night's sleep.

My only option was to try and find foods that caused less of a problem, and then stick to those.

The doctors were somewhat exasperated at my lack of compliance, so suggested a treatment known as Elemental Diet. This was something I had tried in the dim and distant past, so it wasn't unknown to me. Since I remembered it being quite helpful back when I'd had it previously, I agreed to the idea. My mental process surrounding this was that I could use it to settle down whatever inflammation was present, and then I could get a bit further ahead with my own food choices.

Throughout all of this time, I was taking a variety of vitamins and minerals at high doses, based on my underlying idea that if

I could get all the nutrients into my body that it needed to heal itself, then it would begin to do just that.

Anyway, after the doctor's suggestion and my agreement to a course of Elemental Diet, it was a full year before I got to see a dietitian. I've got two things to mention regarding this state of affairs.

First, it proves that in the immediate aftermath of the pandemic response, the health service was no longer functioning in any meaningful way. Having to wait a full year to begin treatment for something considered to be a serious risk is simply not good enough by any measure. This helped confirm to me what I already thought was my only viable option, namely controlling my illness myself without any medical help. I cannot imagine what it must be like to be desperate for treatment yet have to wait so long for it. At least I wasn't desperate to see anyone, instead seeing the idea as little more than a bit of help with what I was already doing.

Second, my understanding about food and my disease expanded considerably over this year, and I am pleased I was given this time, because of what I am about to tell you. If I had not come to my understanding by the time I started with the Elemental Diet, then it may have had a very different outcome, mostly because I would have persevered with it, and I might not be in the position I am today to be able to say I've solved my disease. So, for me at least, a shockingly bad health service turned out in my favour. I finally got an appointment with a dietitian in November 2022.

The day of my appointment was also a day when I had a shift at work. The appointment was quite early, at 11 am, so I went to work very early, at 3 am, with the idea of finishing my shift and getting to the hospital in good time. All was going well with this plan, but at just after 10 am, with only 2 deliveries to go, my van decided to get itself a puncture. I'm not sure if I should classify myself as a superstitious thinker, but I did wonder if the universe was trying to tell me something when this happened. However, in keeping with my default response to little intuitions like this, I chose not to take heed of it.

Changing a wheel on a fairly big van isn't the easiest thing in the world, especially as vehicle manufacturers provide you with a completely inadequate wheel brace and equally ropey-looking jack to carry out such a repair with. It would challenge anyone to loosen a wheel nut tightened to over 200 Newton metres of torque via the tool supplied with the van – a short, angled bar with a socket on the end that is too big for the wheel nut and keeps either slipping off or rounding the corners on the nut. But I had an appointment for 11 am, and I hate to miss appointments, so I directed all the will I could muster into my task and had the punctured wheel off and the spare wheel on within twenty minutes. I arrived at the hospital with hands and face covered in dirt and brake dust, with just minutes to spare.

So, still covered in dirt, I went in to speak to the dietitian. We discussed a bit about food, had some differences of opinion regarding it, and then I left with a prescription for six weeks' worth of elemental drinks.

After a few days of organising supplies, I got started, aiming to stick with it for the full six weeks. In my mind, I thought it would be a chance for a good rest for my endlessly distressed bowel. I also thought it would be good to save a bit of money on the weekly shopping and would free up a bit of time from having to cook anything.

The first few days went reasonably – it's not the easiest thing in the world to stop eating all food and stop drinking all drinks except water, but my memory of it told me that it was going to be helpful, so I managed OK for these first few days.

I have to point out that the taste of the Elemental Diet is something to behold. It smells more like something you would expect to find in a condemned chemical factory as opposed to anything edible or drinkable, and it tastes just about as bad.

One of the strange effects I've always found with these drinks is that initially, they make your insides feel very strange. The best description I can offer is that it feels like you are digesting something with the properties of both rubber and sandpaper at the same time. When I had done this in the past, I would get that feeling for a couple of days, before it subsided and all became calm for the remaining course of the treatment. What this is though is a great big warning that you are doing something wrong.

The rubbery, sandpaper feeling came along right on cue, so I didn't worry too much. However, rather than getting better, it just kept getting worse. About a week in, I was in a whole world of pain, and I was getting shivery, achy feelings more associated with flu, but without the coughing and sneezing. I continued for a couple more days, thinking that maybe it was some healing process underway. However, I began to wonder if I should stop when I started feeling even more unwell.

I decided to read the ingredients that make up the Elemental Diet. I should have done this before starting it, but institutionalisation and the associated trust in professionals is a very difficult thing to step away from, even when you don't have much trust left for them. Elemental drinks are presented as, or perhaps it would be better to say marketed as a cutting-edge technical solution to bowel disease. This had the effect of leading me to believe that I would not be able to glean much from the information sheet, which led to me agreeing to it on faith alone. Upon investigation, however, I discovered several red flags.

The iron in the drinks is in the form of Ferrous Sulphate. There was a time when I could take iron tablets made of this and not suffer any noticeable ill effects from doing so. I was on a high dose of prednisolone at the same time though, and that might be why I didn't experience any negative effects. Not because prednisolone is a solution to anything, but because it short circuits your response to threats and dangers, and you don't get any biofeedback about the damage you are causing to yourself. As time has passed, I've found myself suffering more and more problems with iron supplements. Ferrous Sulphate in particular, even trace amounts of it, causes a lot of pain and digestive discomfort. If I take any, for a few days it seems fine, after which I get stomach pains. These only get worse if I keep taking it, and I rapidly reach a point where I cannot eat anything. This is even if I take the amounts found in multivitamins or in tonics, which is around 14 milligrams a day, compared to around 600 milligrams at prescription levels.

I can draw on direct evidence of what Ferrous Sulphate does to me, along with direct evidence that I can stop the problems it causes by removing it entirely from my diet. I also know that even at levels below the recommended daily allowance, it still causes a whole world of issues in me. Because of this, I stopped the treatment immediately.

After water, the two main ingredients are maltodextrin and sugar. Maltodextrin is a bit iffy, to say the least. Here are a couple of studies if you want a bit more background.

The first is this one...

Crohn's Disease-Associated Adherent-Invasive Escherichia coli Adhesion Is Enhanced by Exposure to the Ubiquitous Dietary Polysaccharide Maltodextrin | PLOS ONE
https://journals.plos.org/plosone/article?id=10.1371/journal.pone.0052132

The other is this one...

Impact of Food Additives on Gut Homeostasis - PMC (nih.gov)
https://www.ncbi.nlm.nih.gov/pmc/articles/PMC6835893/

Maltodextrin is heavily implicated in the development of digestive inflammation. It is one of the few environmental things (environment in the context of the environment of the digestive system) where articles and research directly mention the increased prevalence of Crohn's concerning it.

A side issue of maltodextrin is that it causes a much more pronounced blood sugar spike than normal sugar. So not good if you are looking to avoid diabetic incidents. Even just on this front, the only reason I can see for it being classed as safe is because it is cheap to produce and is of great benefit to the manufacturing and marketing of processed food. It is classed as a complex carbohydrate, so manufacturers can specify lower levels of sugars in ingredients if they use maltodextrin, even though the very same products have a more pronounced sugar effect once ingested than plain and simple sugar would.

In terms of my specific situation, the basic premise of the above two articles is that additives such as maltodextrin affect the mucous lining that protects the epithelial cells of the digestive system (the semi-permeable layer that is the barrier between food passing through the gut and the insides of the body). As far as I can gather, it promotes a separation of the mucous lining from the epithelial cells the mucous is there to protect, leaving the cells open to irritation and damage. Then the resulting ulceration and inflammation that is called Crohn's can develop. So obviously, the best way of treating such a disease is to introduce a far more concentrated form of the thing that might be causing it!

This damage to the protective mucous layer is what I am connecting to the sandpaper/rubber feeling I would always feel when embarking on a course of Elemental Diet. Whether this is the case or not, the studies seem to suggest these drinks are setting up the very conditions required for more inflammation to develop.

Next is sugar, and I'm not going to go too far on this one. The media constantly tells us that sugar is the devil in white granule form. I don't see it as being anywhere near as bad as we are constantly told, as long as it isn't eaten to excess, but the issue I have with it in terms of the Elemental Diet is that it requires digestion to be able to absorb it. Not much, but it needs to be broken down into glucose and fructose before it can be absorbed. So that's a bit strange considering the point of Elemental Diet is to give the digestion a total rest. Maltodextrin is similar in this respect, as it must be broken down into glucose molecules before it can be absorbed.

I'm not going to give you any links to articles or research regarding sugar and inflammation, and this is in large part because I don't see any link in terms of myself. If you do a quick search you'll find the internet is awash with negative stuff regarding it. Be mindful though that sugar is relatively natural when compared to other fillers and bulking agents, and the negative impacts are probably more related to over-indulgence rather than outright toxicity. If sugar was the only ingredient of the elemental drinks that I had flagged up as potentially problematic, I would have probably continued with them.

Next is aspartame. One of the maltodextrin studies I mentioned above has plenty in it about aspartame as well, none of it good for digestive health, with much the same impact as maltodextrin for similar reasons related to the way it affects the mucous membrane.

Maltodextrin has for many years ranked quite high in terms of my understanding of things that aren't good. There was a time (well, many times really) in the past when I was desperately underweight. So I was very often prescribed supplements to boost my calorie intake. I have tried to do process of elimination type exercises many times to try and find out what is causing my problems, and usually give up because I conclude that food in general is the problem. However, maltodextrin, which is the main ingredient of most nutritional supplements given out by the NHS, came out at the top of my lists several times, as I did seem to get worse when ingesting it, even though the extra calories and other nutrients in the supplements should have given me a boost. I even brought this to the attention of doctors, trying more than once to convince them that maltodextrin was making my condition worse, but didn't get far. In the end, I gave up trying to convince anyone about this and went with the assumption that the roots of my problems were unknowable. With hindsight, I think that I have probably identified many of the things that cause me trouble and have done this several times, but I've always approached it via a method of trying to isolate one causative factor. If there is more than one, then my findings usually appear to become invalid after a time.

Why maltodextrin is considered a good thing to give in

concentrated form to someone with Crohn's is now a complete mystery to me. Assuming the research from respected medical bodies such as the NIH (US National Institutes of Health) is indeed correct, then the more you look into this, the more you start to think it is like prescribing cigarettes to someone with lung disease.

As to why the Elemental Diet appears to induce remission is another good question. I'm just theorising here, but perhaps it has to do with the removal of direct irritants (the indigestible bits of stuff in normal food), coupled with the reduced requirement for digestive juices to break things down. A reduction in acidity will mean less general irritation of already inflamed areas. Since the actual irritants are also temporarily removed from the equation, then the protective function of your mucous membrane is not required, since there are no particles for it to block, meaning the body, or more specifically the blood has nothing to respond to (i.e. no particles getting where they shouldn't), and as such can pull back on its assault against whatever it sees as a problem. This will lead to improved results on markers in blood tests, and as such might lead to the assumption that the treatment has indeed induced a remission of the disease, even though it has potentially just caused more damage to the very thing that will protect you once you return to normal food.

To put this into a bit more context, you have to look at what is considered to be the disease. Medical people see the disease as the inflammation itself and therefore occupy themselves with getting rid of that inflammation. If a course of Elemental Diet shows a reduction in that inflammation then it is said to have been a success.

If you flip your thinking around though, and start to look

at the inflammation as being your body doing exactly what it should be doing, namely containing damage and eliminating toxins, then your view of the disease changes completely. Doing this also means you can start looking for what is causing your problems, and then make changes in your life to overcome it. People who profess to be experts in whatever they claim to be an expert in are probably not going to help too much in many cases, as expertise often reduces to broad generalisations about how to improve specific markers in blood tests, regardless of whatever deeper knowledge comes with that expertise. One reason for this probably has to do with how the health system is set up. An appointment with a doctor is at most, ten minutes. Over this time, they have to find out what your problems are, and then come up with a means of alleviating them. Then they have to do the same thing for dozens more people. There is no possibility of doing anything more than prescribing a medicine to improve the immediate expression of an issue. The health service is focused on kicking cans down the road - the only problem is that it will eventually kick all of those cans into a great big heap of cans, and from that point, all it can do is keep nudging the ever-expanding heap along that road.

In terms of Elemental Diet, my above reasoning would seem to indicate that while it may offer temporary relief, it might also lay the seeds for much more disease at a later date, namely because all of that maltodextrin is potentially going to remove even more of the protective mucous lining from your bowel, and leave it open to a great deal more damage as soon as food is re-introduced.

When I started writing this, I had the idea that the solutions being offered to my problems are the cause of more of the very problems they are proposing to solve. I hadn't gone down the Elemental Diet rabbit hole at that point and honestly didn't believe it was yet another instance of this. Now though, and with some surprise, I see it as being the same as all the other pharmaceuticals, in that while it seems to offer an actual solution, it appears to me that it causes more of the problem it is prescribed to solve.

After this episode, the doctors haven't come back to me with any further offers of treatment, other than occasional offers of monoclonal antibodies. Once I got myself settled down from the effects of the drinks, and began to apply the full range of nutrition-based management I was beginning to grasp, my disease just went away all by itself, and the associated markers in my blood stopped flagging up any problems. So the medical people have kind of stepped off the case.

This brings me to the end of my long and convoluted story of how Crohn's disease affected me. In the next chapter, I'll dig a bit deeper into my understanding of the mechanisms behind drug-based treatments, and the chapter after that will explain in a lot more detail the dietary choices that have made a complete difference to me.

7

Medical Mismanagement

I am about to present my understanding of two of the main pharmaceutical products I was prescribed to manage my disease but made it worse as far as I can see. At the end I'll also give you a summary of some of the other prescription drugs on offer, ones I was usually too frightened to take, so never took for long enough to build up any direct picture of what they do.

The drugs I'm going to go into more detail on are prednisolone and omeprazole. With prednisolone, I took varying doses constantly from 1987 for about ten years, and then occasional short courses for another twenty years or so after that. I took omeprazole from around the year 2000, every day until mid-2021, so more than twenty years. I need to point out that the manufacturers only recommend short-term usage of these, so the effects I am talking about are a long way outside of the intended usage scenarios or any safety data.

I'll just remind you that I am not qualified in anything related to medicine, so you must weigh up what I will be saying against the official medical stance regarding these products. I am qualified to talk about computer software development though, which might not seem immediately relevant, but please bear with me here. I'm going to tell you a bit about how a computer programmer might build up a picture of a system to construct a software model of it, and this is something that has a great deal of relevance when it comes to analysing and organising other fields of knowledge.

Before I explain how a software developer might produce a model, I'll tell you about the flip side of good code design, and explain one of the ways the whole process can go awry. One of the quirks of writing a computer program is that if you get something wrong, you aren't necessarily stopped in your tracks straight away. You can go on building, patching over and around your mistakes for a considerable distance beyond them. You can even convince yourself that you didn't make any mistakes and that it is just the complex nature of your task making things so difficult. But there always comes a point where the increasing complexity of your patching and bypassing efforts will slow your progress to something resembling a standstill. Instead of moving forward, you end up in the programming equivalent of wading through mud.

When you end up in this mud, you are all too aware of the difficulty you endured to get there, so you are loath to give up and start again. You will go to extreme lengths to keep pushing through, shoehorning more and more code into the program just to hold it together, no matter how thick the mud gets or how much it weighs you down. You might also get to prove to yourself just how clever you are by navigating around your mistakes and holding your algorithmic mess together for whatever code you are writing, but the result will be a bug-ridden nightmare to understand and maintain (and I will go as far as to say this is probably a feature of the vast majority of software in existence).

I have more than a strong suspicion that most scientific endeavours have a susceptibility towards similar problems. Perhaps this wasn't always the case, mainly because science was originally concerned with the engineering of actual machines that either worked or didn't. The modern shift into unseen realms has created some fertile ground for fundamental errors, ones that can then be endlessly patched over and around to hold a faulty hypothesis together.

Now for something that does explain a bit about software development, and this is the concept of modelling, with particular reference to physical and logical models. If you go online and look up physical and logical models in terms of computing, you will find yourself reading about databases, along with the nuances of how the computer stores the data as opposed to how the developer designs the data structures. The kind of programming I used to do wasn't concerned with databases, but I found it very helpful to apply the concepts of physical and logical models to the code itself (meaning what I am about to describe might seem different to the textbook explanations if you decide to go and fact-check me, but the principle is the same).

The starting point of any project is a perceptual idea of what is required, which can also be described as a logical model. In simpler terms, it's a definition of what you want the computer to do. Computers work a bit differently to a human mind though, so to get a computer to do what you want, you have to convert your initial model into a form a machine can work with. This is what programming is, and you can describe the resulting code as a physical model. A physical model is an accurate representation of what is going on inside the machine, so, at the absolute lowest level, is concerned with electricity flowing through constantly adapting circuits. This doesn't make much sense to anyone though (other than electronic engineers and physicists), so the concept of a physical model expands to mean an accurate representation of how data is stored and manipulated inside the computer. However, even this can be of very little use when it comes to developing some code to perform a computing task, as it often doesn't provide all that much in the way of meaning, hence the need for a logical model to work from. It might be more illuminating to say perceptual rather than logical though, as there is a bit of ambiguity in the minds of some non-computing types as to what logical means in the context I am using here.

Going back to the starting point of any software project, you begin with a general idea of what you want the computer to do. From there, you magnify your idea into components. You then look at each component, magnifying each one into sub-components, and then go into each of these, continually magnifying each distinct part of each one, slowly building up the overall structure of the program. This can be described as a logical structure or model for the final code. Eventually, you reach a point where you can define the individual steps of what you are doing in terms of pure mathematical logic, meaning you can specify code flow in terms of things either being true or false. Once you arrive at such a point, you can write some actual code inside the overall structure, and this can be perceived as a physical code model. However, computers work on the principle of layers, and as such, even the final code you write can be viewed as another logical model. It still has to be compiled into machine code before the computer will run it (and then the machine code further reduces down to microcode and beyond), but from the perspective of programming, it can be seen as the physical implementation of the original logic.

The job of a systems analyst, in the context of software development, is to produce a logical model of whatever real-world process is to be simulated in a computer program, and to do this he or she must be able to quickly identify and then organise the relevant parts of any specialism into a working structure, which can then be used to produce a code implementation of whatever the process under scrutiny happens to be. Back when I did programming there was a great deal of cross-over between programming and analysis. It's been a while since I've done any though, so maybe there is more of a difference these days.

A good analyst can define any system with just enough specificity to enable a computer program to either mimic, integrate with, or take control of that system. Unnecessarily complex definitions lead to more potential for bugs and errors in code (and errors increase exponentially as complexity increases), whereas overly simple definitions lead to incomplete or inaccurate software implementations. So a big part of the job of analysis is to recognise what is important to the task at hand as well as discard whatever is not.

The reason I've explained all of this is because I'm about to construct models of what is going on with the medications I'm looking at, and need to head off the potential for accusations of not being able to do so. I will warn you though, that systems modelling is not always a linear process. Often, several different areas of knowledge must be pulled into the model as it is being constructed, so please bear with me if I appear to be jumping in and out of different subject areas as I go. This is one of the key but largely unrecognised skills required for software development.

So, before looking at what certain drugs do, it might be useful to specify some relevant parts of the digestive process. While I might be glossing over or even skipping a whole lot of detail, it is accurate enough and detailed enough to work with when I come to explain the effects of the drugs I'm discussing.

OK, starting with food on a plate, or in a bowl, or some other container, you put pieces of it in your mouth. Once you have some in your mouth, you chew it to mush it up and mix it with a bit of saliva, thus making it wet and soft and slippery enough to be able to swallow it. It goes down your throat to your stomach, which secretes hydrochloric acid (Hydrogen Chloride in aqueous form, meaning dissolved in water), so this gets added into the mix. The stomach also releases pepsinogen, a precursor to pepsin. Pepsin is an enzyme that breaks proteins down into amino acids, and hydrochloric acid turns pepsinogen into pepsin. Another way of saying this is that the acid activates protein-digesting enzymes. This mixture then passes through your duodenum and into your small bowel, where bile is also mixed into it, and bile is there to break fats down. All the way along, a range of additional digestive enzymes are also secreted into the mix, starting in the mouth and continuing throughout the small bowel. The bile and the enzymes break food down into nutrients that can be absorbed into the bloodstream, and this absorption occurs in the small bowel, via a semi-permeable membrane known as the epithelial layer. This is a layer of cells, only one cell thick, that will allow molecules up to a certain size to pass through, but not any larger ones, hence the need for the bile and the enzymes to break food constituents down into pieces small enough to pass through that barrier. The digestive tract also maintains a layer of mucous to lubricate the stuff passing through it, and to protect the epithelial layer, which as I just mentioned is only one cell thick and is the only other barrier between your bloodstream and whatever you have put in your mouth and swallowed. Anyway, once this mix gets through your small bowel, the nutrients made available by the enzymes and bile have been extracted, and the rest arrives at your large bowel, or colon, as a wet and sloppy liquid. Your colon then reabsorbs the water from this and packs what remains into smelly brown lumps that you drop off into a toilet when required. At least this is what happens if all is going well.

Just to be clear, I'll also specify what an ulcer is, and what inflammation is. Here is the first sentence of an official definition of an ulcer...

"In general, an ulcer is any eroded area of skin or a mucous membrane, marked by tissue disintegration."

https://www.encyclopedia.com/medicine/diseases-and-condit ions/pathology/ulcer

So, and this is very important to understand, an ulcer is a missing bit of tissue or mucous membrane. It is where some part of you has died off or disappeared, so it is a gap or a hole in whatever is supposed to be there, meaning the ulcer is what isn't there, rather than something that is there. For the longest time, I thought an ulcer was basically the same thing as inflammation, and therefore something that affected cells while those cells were still in situ and alive. However, an ulcer should be considered as being a disappearance of something.

Inflammation, on the other hand, is swelling around the site of some damage or something that might be a threat to the body. The purpose of inflammation is to contain damage by stopping it from spreading and to provide resources to enable repairs. It will surround an area of ulceration, toxicity, or injury, and will attempt to bring with it the raw materials required for repairing or removing whatever the problem is.

There is no minimum size requirement for an ulcer to be defined as an ulcer. Therefore, any amount of disintegration is an ulcer, whether that covers an area measured in the number of missing cells, a distance of centimetres, or any other dimension you can think of. The same is true of inflammation. Any amount of it is inflammation, not just when it reaches a certain size. However, since inflammation has the basic property of swelling, given an equivalent amount of ulceration and inflammation, the inflammation will be more readily identifiable. The point here is that if the body responds to some developing ulceration by surrounding it with inflammation, the inflammation will become visible long before the ulceration it is trying to contain.

OK, so keeping in mind these definitions of ulcers and inflammation, and the above model of the digestive process, let's first look at what prednisolone is doing in terms of its use as a treatment for inflammatory bowel disease.

Prednisolone mimics cortisol, and cortisol is a hormone released by the adrenal glands, but this statement doesn't mean much unless you know about hormones and what they do. The full answer to what hormones do would be a very long one, but for what I need to explain about prednisolone I can keep it quite brief.

To understand the function of hormones in the context required here, I'll first explain a bit about the nervous system. In white coat land, the nervous system is organised into a hierarchy, and it is taught to prospective future brainboxes as being factual. However, I contend that the knowledge base surrounding the nervous system is nothing other than an example of a logical model.

The nervous system has to do with the flow of electricity through the body. Of further interest, not really relevant to where I am going, but interesting enough for me to add here is the subject of what people consider life to be. Materialism, which is the foundation of modern science, would have us believe that life is a biological process and that all the electrical stuff going on in a living being is merely a by-product, or maybe a subset of the function of biology. I can think of a very good argument for it being the other way around though, namely that biology is very much secondary to electricity in terms of what being alive is. Consider the moment of death in a person or other living thing and ask yourself what is it that disappears in that moment. It is the electricity that dissipates, not the biological matter suddenly evaporating. Based on this simple fact, it should be obvious that life is an electrical process, meaning biology is just the container for the life that takes up residence in it. Add to this the basic principle that energy cannot be lost, merely changed from one form to another, along with the fact that electricity is a form of energy, and you can then start to understand that the electrical you has existed for the whole of time up to now, will exist for the whole of time yet to come, and as such death can be considered as simply moving out of your body, not ceasing to exist. I can't say whether this electricity stays together, or whether it takes your life experiences and memories along with it, but I can say it still exists in some form.

Anyway, putting aside the meaning of life, the accepted model of the nervous system is split into two major areas of circuitry, the central nervous system and the peripheral nervous system.

The central nervous system consists of the brain and spinal cord, and the peripheral nervous system consists of everything that isn't the brain and spinal cord. The peripheral nervous system is further split into the somatic nervous system and the autonomic nervous system.

The somatic nervous system is the bit we have awareness of and conscious control over, so this includes inputs via our senses and intentional movements via our muscles. This is where our day-to-day awareness resides.

The autonomic nervous system is more of an autopilot feature. It controls the functioning of internal organs, heartbeat, breathing, and digestion. We do get some conscious control over parts of this, most obviously breathing, but the autonomic nervous system will keep everything running when we are busy doing more interesting things.

The autonomic nervous system is further split into the sympathetic nervous system, the parasympathetic nervous system, and the enteric nervous system. The enteric nervous system controls our digestion, and even though I am writing a book about digestive issues, I'm not going to mention the enteric system much more.

The sympathetic and parasympathetic nervous systems are concerned with regulating our responses to our immediate environment. The official description of these is that the sympathetic nervous system activates our fight or flight response, whereas the parasympathetic nervous system returns the body to a relaxed, calm state. We are just about getting to hormones here.

The way the sympathetic and parasympathetic systems control different states in the body is by controlling the release of hormones into the bloodstream. The purpose of hormones is to induce physiological changes so the body can adapt to whatever the current situation requires of it. You could say they act as a bridge between the physical body and the electrical being. Hormones are released by various glands in the body, but for this discussion, we don't need to go that far, apart from saying that the nervous system will stimulate different glands via electrical signals as and when required.

I'm going to diverge a bit from the scientific explanation of these parts of the nervous system now. This is because I am not trying to recreate the scientific model of the nervous system as such, just drawing some required information from it. At the level of understanding I am explaining here, there is an implication that the sympathetic and parasympathetic systems are mutually exclusive, meaning you might jump to a binary conclusion regarding them. I do know that in terms of a deeper scientific analysis, this is not the case, but it might seem so when just scratching the surface.

For the current purposes, it is essential to see the sympathetic and parasympathetic systems as being an analogue system, meaning a sliding scale with extremes at either end, rather than a binary system where only one or the other is switched on at any one time. Also, the words sympathetic and parasympathetic don't speak much in terms of meaning.

So, let's discard all the big words, and redefine what it is alluding to by describing it as a sliding scale of a person's state of being, using the words 'active' and 'passive', with fully active at one end and fully passive at the other. Just to clarify what I mean, I'll give you two examples, each of which might induce a state towards one end of the active–passive scale I have just flagrantly invented.

Imagine you were walking in the woods and you came across

a lost bear cub, then turned to find that mother bear, feeling very angry due to having lost her baby, had recently located her lost cub, but you were now standing in between mother and cub, and mother bear was extremely displeased by this turn of events. In such a situation you would most probably enter into a fully active state.

If, on the other hand, you were sitting in a lecture hall, listening to some boring teacher droning on in a monotone voice about the finer points of databases, then you might enter into a fully passive state.

I've never been in the lost bear cub in the woods situation, but have been in the boring database lecture, so can state with some confidence, that one does induce a passive state, which is another way of saying I struggled tremendously to stay awake. I think it is fair to assume that coming between a mother bear and her cub would induce a completely active state.

To enter a fully active state, also known as fight or flight, the nervous system stimulates the adrenal glands to release adrenaline and cortisol. An online search about either of these hormones will give you a whole lot of very detailed information, along with a considerable amount of fluff.

There is perhaps more to it than what I am going to describe, but at the most basic level, cortisol triggers the release of glucose from cells into the bloodstream, and adrenaline prevents glucose from being removed from the bloodstream and returned to the cells, by blocking the release of insulin. So when people talk about an adrenaline rush, what they mean is a great big sugar rush. The digestive process, or the enteric nervous system, also shuts down during such situations, possibly due to a lack of glucose to power all the little internal muscle contractions required to make the digestive system work.

Without going too far into all the intricacies of metabolism, glucose is the basic fuel element in our bodies. In a fully active, or fight or flight situation, all available energy is required for the immediate situation, so the dual action of cortisol and adrenaline is to pull glucose from cells into the bloodstream, and prevent cells from taking that glucose back from the blood.

Now then, the point of what I am getting to, while not to give you a full explanation of the hormonal system, otherwise known as the endocrine system, is to show why prednisolone is not a good solution to an inflammatory disease.

So, with the information I've presented so far, it should seem fair to assume that increased levels of cortisol/prednisolone are going to push your state towards the active end of the active–passive scale I am framing this in terms of, as it is going to maintain more glucose in your blood than would be there without the cortisol. To do such a thing, glucose is taken from the cells, leaving cells with a deficit of the glucose they ideally need.

I have plenty of experience with the effects of taking prednisolone, and it certainly does support this assumption. One of the main effects I found was increased energy levels, nudging towards the realms of being high on stimulants. In addition, it promoted a general feeling of extreme wellness.

If you decide to learn a bit more about cortisol, you will find that it is known to reduce inflammation, hence the use of prednisolone as an anti-inflammatory medication. As with a lot of what I am writing about, I need to clarify my stance here. I am not saying there should never be a case for using it. In an acute situation, it can quite literally be lifesaving. However, its use as an ongoing solution to chronic inflammation is a really bad idea, for reasons I'm about to get to. Most doctors do agree with this, so I'm broadly on the same page as medical people here.

The next question is regarding the anti-inflammatory effect. Whenever I have asked doctors, the answers tend to have been rather ambiguous explanations regarding immune suppression, or the dampening of my allegedly faulty immune system. This implies that my immune system is a tangible thing, much like an arm or a leg. It is rather difficult to locate the boundaries of an immune system though, so it might be better to view the immune system as yet another logical model.

I'm going to postulate that the anti-inflammatory effect attributed to cortisol is more related to the simple mechanism of it stealing energy from cells and reassigning that energy into the bloodstream, meaning cells don't have the required energy to perform their normal functions. Maybe this is how medical experts already understand things, but if they do then it is not how they explain it to normal people. Normal people are just told that prednisolone reduces inflammation. In terms of the fight or flight response, it is well known that entering into fight or flight mode stops the body from performing its self-healing functions, so my claim here is that the fuel to perform these is simply not available, rather than there being any higher intelligence behind it.

There is also a general idea that cortisol reduces stress. Again, this is usually presented in rather ambiguous terms. Reducing it down into more simple terms, we feel good, at least for a while, when we eat sugar, and this good feeling is the opposite of a stressed feeling, which can be defined as not feeling good. An example of a guaranteed path to stress is the result we feel if we don't have the energy to do all of the things we need to do, yet we still have to do them. Given a set of circumstances, whether or not you feel stressed by them comes down to whether you feel as if you have enough energy to manage them. Having extra glucose in your blood is going to help with your immediate energy demands, meaning an increase in cortisol leading to an increase in blood sugar is going to help prevent feelings of stress, simply because you have additional energy to meet the immediate demands you are under.

The reason I have replaced sympathetic and parasympathetic with an active-passive scale and have described your state as a point between the two extremes is that the ideal state to be in most of the time is somewhere in the middle, meaning you are alert enough to function but also relaxed enough to digest your food and heal damaged parts of your body. So, finally, I'm about up to where I was going concerning the use of prednisolone to suppress inflammation.

Having been under the impression for a long time that the inflammation was my disease, I now see it as having been my body's natural healing mechanism, stimulated to contain whatever the actual problem was. Granted, this swelling caused blockages in my digestive system which led to all of the problems associated with the disease, but I am convinced that the inflammation was nothing more than a response to underlying damage.

I have been told many times that the cause of the inflammation cannot be pinpointed, hence the medical community's uncertainty about what causes Crohn's. Maybe this is because they are looking for an actual thing, and coming to the conclusion that since they cannot find that thing, there must be some other reason for inflammation being triggered, such as a faulty immune system. However, if you are looking for something, this means you are going to pass right over places where there isn't anything, and remembering the earlier definition of an ulcer, you are not necessarily in the correct mental place to recognise the absence of something as being the thing you are looking for. You are more likely to look to the edges of that space in your search for the thing you are looking for, and in cases such as mine, you are going to find inflammation with no apparent reason for being there, particularly if the inflammation is visible but many of the areas of ulceration it is responding to are too small to be seen. Medical science, having been unable to find damage or a specific pathogen to blame, looks instead for a genetic reason, and busies itself in the meantime with reducing the associated inflammation.

Now then, an increased level of cortisol or prednisolone is going to take glucose away from cells that would otherwise be performing the task of containing and trying to heal areas of ulceration, meaning the inflammation is going to reduce since the energy is not there to maintain it. This means ulceration isn't going to have any chance to heal, and as such it is much more likely to spread further. However, since the inflammation has reduced, this will result in an improvement in immediate symptoms, and diagnostic tests will confirm the reduction in inflammation, leading to a false positive conclusion that the medication has promoted an improvement in the underlying condition.

I'll say this one more time. Prednisolone steals energy from cells and gives it to the blood, making you feel more energetic and less stressed. Because energy is being taken out of the cells, those cells no longer have enough energy to perform actual healing actions, such as containing and repairing damage, so the damage is left unattended, leaving it free to spread further. As to what causes this damage, take your pick from general irritants, poisoning, malnutrition, or a combination.

If you remember back to somewhere near the start of the book, I claimed that prednisolone seemed to cause more disease in me, while helping with the immediate symptoms, and that there was a big can of worms to open regarding it. The explanation I have put forward here hopefully gets through a least a few of the worms in that particular can.

So that is my assessment of why prednisolone causes more of the disease it is used as a solution for. It is mostly just used as a temporary fix now, but when I was first diagnosed it was more common as an ongoing solution (however, when framing something as a temporary fix, there is still a need to factor in the cumulative effect, and how often it is used temporarily).

Next up is omeprazole, or any other proton pump inhibitor for that matter, meaning drugs that reduce the amount of acid being secreted by the lining of the stomach.

To understand the effect on the digestive system of reduced stomach acid, it is probably a good idea to get acquainted with the purpose of acid, and therefore the reasons why it is there in the first place.

A quick online search will tell you it is essential to break down food to aid digestion. This is presented as a fact. I've asked several gastroenterologists this very question and they seem a bit less certain than the internet does, giving rather more ambiguous answers, although perhaps they are unable to describe the functions of acid in layman's terms, so opt to give vague answers to their patients instead. I haven't asked about this for many years, so a gastric doctor might give you a more detailed and complete explanation today.

Aside from breaking down food, I've read some claims that

acid has something to do with killing bugs and parasites. Modern living, with its quest for cleanliness and all things sterile, could mask whether it makes much difference in this area, though. Another stated function of acid is to stimulate the release of bile and more digestive enzymes. As with the bugs and parasites concept, I can't give you any further insight into this, other than saying it would seem reasonable to assume that when the stomach is full of food and acid is being secreted, it would be useful if the full range of digestive juices were also released into the digestive system, to break down all the components of that food. I don't know if this is the case, or if the other digestive juices have completely independent methods of having their release stimulated, so I'm not about to make any claims in this area.

One thing I can state as an absolute fact is that the presence of acid in the stomach is a natural or default condition of the digestive process. A bit of a statement of the obvious, but there is no ambiguity to it, so it is factual.

Building on this, the internet is fairly certain that gastric acid will activate protein-digesting enzymes, meaning it will react with the pepsinogen that is also secreted by the stomach wall, turning it into pepsin, which can break proteins down into amino acids, and those can be absorbed into the bloodstream as building blocks for the body to make its proteins.

There is also a much-repeated claim online that stomach acid helps with the absorption of minerals, but generally without much context as to why this is the case, so maybe I can help with a bit of explanation. Feel free to skip this next couple of paragraphs if you just want to take my word, and the internet's word for it, but here is why acid helps with mineral absorption.

Looking at basic chemical properties, acids help to dissolve things, so it would seem fairly safe to assume that stomach acid is there to perform some sort of similar function with the food it comes into contact with. The term 'dissolve' is where a substance, whatever that may be, gets mixed with water and disappears into that water. It will find an easier path to becoming dissolved when there is acid present in the water. I don't want to go too far into Chemistry to explain, as I'm not writing a Chemistry textbook, but in chemical terms, all atoms (or elements) are looking to exist in a stable form. This stability is defined as an atom having a full outer shell of electrons. You'll have to look up what I mean by shells of electrons elsewhere if you don't understand the theory of them. Molecules, which are combinations of atoms, can be perceived as elements either donating or receiving electrons to and from one another. Stable molecules form when different atoms stick together to facilitate this electron sharing.

Ionic molecules are defined as simple combinations, where a metal with a natural surplus of electrons donates these electrons to an element or a combination of elements with a natural deficit of electrons. Then the metal, and whatever it is bound to, stick together and form a stable molecule. When such a molecule is added to water, the bond holding the positive and negative parts together can break apart, allowing the metal and the non-metal part to dissolve independently into the water, and these parts are called ions (hence the name ionic molecules) – the metal ion has a positive charge, and the non-metal part has a negative charge, and this is because the negative part keeps the electrons donated by the metal part when the molecule formed. When there is acid in water, what this means is that the water contains positively charged hydrogen ions (in the case of hydrochloric acid, the water also contains negatively charged chloride ions, but hydrogen is the particle of interest here). Hydrogen is the smallest element that exists, and as such a positive hydrogen ion has the biggest possible ratio of charge in terms of how positive that positive charge is. Since it is missing the single electron it once possessed, it is entirely positively charged, and this is more positive in relative terms than any other ion can be. This makes hydrogen ions much more reactive than any other ion, so when an ionic type of molecule is added to acidified water, the non-metal part of that molecule is going to be drawn away from the metal and toward the hydrogen ions in the water, weakening the bonds holding the molecule together, meaning it is going to break apart and dissolve into the water much faster than into plain water.

I could go much further into more detail, as what I have described is missing quite a bit in terms of a full explanation, but if we change some of the words it might become more apparent how this applies to the process of digestion. In the above description, if we change the term 'ionic molecule' to 'metal salt', and then change the words 'metal', and 'non-metal' to 'mineral', we will get right to what the internet tells you about stomach acid making minerals easier to absorb. We could also use the word 'electrolyte' in place of 'mineral' (technically speaking, any ionic molecule turns into electrolytes when dissolved as the water becomes electrically conductive).

So, back to where I was, the food you eat contains minerals, and the acid in your stomach either dissolves, or helps keep them dissolved in water, which allows them to be absorbed into the bloodstream as dissolved ions, or electrolytes. A reduction in acid means this process will occur to a lesser degree, meaning nutrients will not be as readily available for absorption. Additionally, there are potentially going to be more undissolved particles passing through the digestive tract, and these could become irritants rather than the nutrients they should be.

I've already mentioned the action of turning pepsinogen into pepsin, thus starting the process of breaking down protein into amino acids, meaning the protein you eat becomes bioavailable. The same potential case exists for proteins as I mentioned for minerals, whereby proteins that have not been broken down into amino acids are possibly going to become an irritant rather than a nutrient source. So, that gives us two reasons why gastric acid is probably essential to the process of digestion and two reasons why suppressing it long-term could potentially lead to the promotion of additional disease. For a third reason, as well as an increase in irritants, there is going to be more of a tendency towards malnutrition, meaning a potential lack of resources for the body to repair the damage (arguably made worse by the first two reasons), and maintain overall health.

I was initially going to tie conditions of acidity with gut flora, but then I started looking into the subject of gut flora and found myself in a world of circular reasoning. Let me explain, as where I ended up might go against everything you might have read or been told about digestive health.

The basic premise regarding bacteria and digestive health is that there is a symbiotic process going on, where if you have 'good' bacteria populating your digestive system, then this will promote good health. Equally, if you have 'bad' bacteria then this will allegedly lead to problems. The presence of certain bacteria is linked to certain health outcomes, which gives rise to the idea in some circles that bacteria itself is a causative factor in the underlying health of the gut.

The probiotics section of the food industry would certainly have you believe this. The medical industry is kind of on the fence, neither advocating for nor against the idea for the most part, although doctors have prescribed soluble fibre to me in the past, meaning they must accept the principle of probiotics at some level (soluble fibre is considered a food source for 'good' bacteria). The concept of maintaining your good bacteria is a mainstay of various holistic treatments.

So, all in all, the advice seems to indicate that looking after your gut flora is something you should be doing to promote a healthy digestive system. Based on such a premise, it would then seem fairly straightforward to imply that having the right bacteria inside of you is going to be of benefit, hence the widely touted idea that a route to good health is to ingest those good bacteria and thus boost the types that are commonly found in the guts of healthy people.

It is very easy to turn this around though. The function of bacteria, broadly speaking, is to break down dead or inorganic matter. Colonies of bacteria themselves are most probably not in possession of all that much intelligence, and as such will most likely just be looking for food to eat to stay alive and replicate, rather than pondering the reasons for their existence, or making free and informed choices about where to live. Different forms of bacteria have different dietary requirements, and as such it could very easily be argued that the condition of, and content of, the digestive system could be far more important in determining the bacteria that is found there, as opposed to the bacteria in residence being the reason for the underlying health of the system.

A healthy system full of appropriate food, digested as it should be, is going to provide a very different menu to the resident bacteria than one full of junk, or a damaged system that isn't breaking foods down properly. You can throw as much good bacteria into an unhealthy system as you want, but it is not going to thrive in such a system, as there is not going to be anything it can eat and derive sustenance from in that system. The types of bacteria labelled as bad, on the other hand, might simply be finding an endless banquet to chew and chomp their way through.

Medical literature regarding the overall impact of omeprazole is a bit sparse, to say the least. Here's one study though, looking at the observable effect of the medicine on colonic bacteria, if you want to have a look at it...

The effect of omeprazole treatment on the gut microflora and neutrophil function – PubMed (nih.gov)
https://pubmed.ncbi.nlm.nih.gov/28258834/

This was a study of the effect after 4 weeks of treatment. A quote from the conclusion is, "Omeprazole treatment have caused considerable changes in stool culture results. Patients treated with the higher dose had some tendency to decreased diversity of colonic microflora and towards changes in fermenting bacteria of the gut." (grammatical errors as written in the study)

So it does lead to changes in observable flora within the gut, and this happens in quite a short time frame. The study does not indicate whether this effect is due to direct action on the bacteria, whether the change of environmental acidity then promotes the proliferation of different bacteria, whether the removal of acid changes how food is broken down (or not), thus leading to different bacteria gaining an advantage, or whether part of the function of the acid is to kill the very bacteria that take up residence once that acid is no longer there, or anything else in terms of any real insight. However, it does offer proof that suppressing acid production leads to changes in the observable digestive environment. This does not mean that taking probiotics is going to offer any solution, because logic, or at least my version of logic, would seem to suggest that the observed bacteria is very much downstream from the real issues. There are no studies I'm aware of looking at these issues, or at what the effect is long term.

The manufacturers of omeprazole, and all other proton pump inhibitors, only recommend short-term courses, of twelve weeks at most, or thereabouts. I took it for almost 20 years. At the time of writing, cases are starting to make it to court regarding long-term use, but these seem to be centred on kidney damage, something I don't know about, so won't comment on either way.

I've never heard anything linking it to causing or promoting digestive ulceration long-term, but I can't unlearn my direct experience of it, and my direct experience tells me it does just that. I think a combination of reduced nutrient availability along with an increased prevalence of irritants is enough to gradually worsen the overall state of the digestive system. Maybe not over the recommended courses of two or three months, but certainly over many years. However, since no peer-reviewed papers are talking about this, the medical consensus is that I am wrong, and that is that.

I'll reiterate that I'm not holding the manufacturers entirely responsible for my outcome, as they only specify short courses of their product. Therefore taking it for longer periods is outside of the circumstances they state as being safe.

Whether there is any truth or not in my theorising, the fact that omeprazole masks symptoms means you have no conscious way of knowing what is going on with the foods you eat, and that in itself is a major problem. Arguably, yet another very important function of stomach acid is to tell you when you have eaten something you shouldn't have, by giving you indigestion. Under normal circumstances, when you eat something difficult for your system to break down, your stomach will produce more and more acid to try and resolve it, presenting you with plenty of feedback about the effect of what you just ate. You can then take this information on board, and avoid eating whatever caused the indigestion in future. Suppressing the production of acid will prevent indigestion, but means you have no way of building up any picture of what you should and should not be eating.

There's also the question of what happens to the acid-forming chemicals that no longer resolve their existence via a path to acid in your stomach when medicine is taken to prevent it. What I mean by saying this is that the acid that is normally secreted by your stomach is made out of something, and if that something isn't being turned into acid, then it must be either accumulating somewhere, or must be being turned into something else, and neither of these scenarios seem ideal.

Stopping taking omeprazole after so many years is difficult, to say the least. Since it prevents the feedback that would stop you in your tracks much sooner, your system is free to develop wide-ranging problems unchecked. Once you have such problems, gastric acid does become your enemy, as any increase in acid production aggravates the problems. This can lead to some very acute and very life-threatening internal bleeds. So, your life becomes dependent on your continued dosage of the medicine, hence the actions of medical professionals in continuing to prescribe it. The only way to achieve coming off it is very, very slowly. I tried to stop a few times via dose reduction, but as with my earlier steroid experience, I would keep reaching a point where things got so bad I had to go right back up to the full dose, with the knowledge by then that it was possibly causing the very illness that I was taking it for.

Considering prednisolone, and comparing that with omeprazole, there's a pattern developing here, I think. My experience of both is that ultimately, they promote the continuation, and very likely a worsening, of the very disease they are alleviating the symptoms of. Add to this my thoughts regarding the Elemental Diet treatment path, which seems to be yet another case of the treatment causing more of the disease it is treating, and it would appear, at least to me, that the treatments for Crohn's are one of the reasons for it being lifelong and incurable.

I have taken other medications for inflammation, and have briefly mentioned some of them. I never really stuck with them for very long though, so don't have any depth of experience regarding their effects directly, and as such am not well-placed to discuss much more about them. My default position about almost any pharmaceutical medication is that you do not have whatever illness you have because your body is deficient in a chemical that came out of a lab.

I've always been very reticent about these other medicine-based methods of reducing inflammation, due to the potential for catastrophic side effects. Azathioprine / 6MP are classed as chemotherapy drugs, and that in itself is enough for me to have never really given them too much consideration. While the technical meaning of chemotherapy is treatment with any chemical, effectively meaning all medicines, the more usual understanding of it is highly toxic substances that may offer some benefit when facing cancer, something that is going to kill you anyway without drastic action. In such situations, the potential for toxicity-related issues is secondary to the disease. For something like ongoing inflammation though, to me, it has always seemed a very big risk to literally poison the body to control the inflammation. I did try 6MP a few times, but each time I felt rotten after a few months.

The general idea behind 6MP and Azathioprine (they are the same thing once inside of you) is to suppress your body's production of white blood cells, and thus 'dampen' your immune system, leading to a reduction of inflammation. They are not quite as focused as this might make them seem, though. They suppress the function of bone marrow, meaning they reduce the production of red blood cells as well as white ones, and even though I don't know much more about this, it doesn't seem too good of an idea to suppress the production of any blood cells, of whatever colour. As well as the headline side effects of potential lymphomas and/or organ failure, they promote more susceptibility to other infections, and this seems a very big risk to me, especially given the disjointed nature of the health service. If I am on the right lines regarding the reasons why the body produces inflammation, then the result of long-term suppression of it, via whatever method, could also lead to the same kinds of consequences I have outlined for prednisolone, namely that the actual damage could then be left unattended.

Monoclonal antibodies are the other major treatment path in medical settings, and probably the most popular one at present. As with the chemotherapy drugs, I have always considered the potential risks to be far greater than the benefits. I explained my reservations regarding the manufacturing processes in an earlier chapter. For that reason alone, I have never had any confidence in the use of them. In terms of their intended effects, they mostly block the effects of certain proteins in the body, but these proteins, as well as being linked to inflammation, are related to wider immune function.

As with azathioprine and 6MP, this makes a patient much more susceptible to infection, and much less able to fight off such infection. This includes, but is not limited to: colds, urinary tract infections, tuberculosis (but didn't my BCG vaccine solve that?), and sepsis(!). They may increase the risk of developing lymphoma. According to drug information sheets, the potential for lymphoma is unclear, even though it seems to be absolutely clear enough to get a mention on the information leaflet. They might also affect liver function, so patients are advised to keep an eye out for any signs of jaundice. So, all in all, remembering the fact they are extracted from cancerous cells, there's nothing to worry about there.

The one time I did try one of these biologics, it made me feel terrible, in the kind of way I would imagine kidney failure to feel, so I gave up on it very quickly. Aside from this, it wasn't a case of taking a prescription to the chemist and getting the medicine. While this form of treatment is usually done via an intravenous drip at the hospital, the one I tried came in self-injectable syringes, meaning I could take it at home. I agreed to it, then a few days later a bloke turned up in an unmarked van with my supplies. This was because it was under an EUA (Emergency Use Authorisation), meaning it couldn't legally come through regular channels, and this was because there was no real safety profile. Overall, it felt like some kind of dodgy drug deal. After a few doses of it, I got severe lower back pains and thus ended my tryout of monoclonal antibodies.

One other treatment I tried for a while, and almost forgot about, was mesalazine, which is a derivative of salicylic acid, and so in a similar group of chemicals to aspirin. I took it for quite a while, sometime back in the 1990s, as it got the doctors off my back about having to take something. I can't say whether it had any positive effect at all, though. As with all of the available medicines, there is a long list of potential negative outcomes.

One other treatment I was offered, and this was quite recently, was Methotrexate. I considered it but then found you are not supposed to go out in the sun when you take it. That fact alone prevented me from taking it.

That is about the entire repertoire of official treatment options for inflammatory bowel disease. All have significant associated risks.

One other class of pharmaceutical drug I have come into contact with is opioid painkillers. When all else fails, the likes of morphine, codeine, tramadol, and other variations offer some temporary relief. They are more than just a little bit addictive though, and it is very easy to keep taking them long after the pain-killing effect has stopped, and then continue long after the pain itself has ended. As such, they can rapidly become yet another problem to contend with, as opposed to something offering any help.

8

Quality And Quantity

Up to now I've given you a brief history of my disease, and have made considerable effort to explain why I think the available medications are of no help. I need to do something to control my situation, so what is left after medicine?

The most obvious answer to that question is food. Most of us will know of some foods that don't particularly agree with us, and we will also have some level of understanding about how eating certain foods will make us healthier, whereas consuming others will do the opposite. This doesn't imply we will necessarily have the correct or the best understanding, but we all have some sort of knowledge. The messaging relating to healthy and unhealthy choices is relentless, so even if we don't follow what we are told is in our best interests, it is difficult to remain unaware of the existence of good and bad dietary choices, whatever they may turn out to be.

I could fill a bookshelf with books about how to cure Crohn's via nutrition, and could easily fill an entire bookcase if looking at disease in general. I'm not going to comment on diseases beyond my own because they have nothing to do with me, and

I'm not even going to say much of anything about the books and articles related to inflammatory bowel disease.

There have been times when I tried following the directions of various sources of information related to my illness, as well as many more regarding health and wellness in general. None ever really worked for me.

I never managed to stick to any diet plan from such sources. Partly, this is because they tend to require something of an approach of military precision. Also, they tend to involve eating foods that I don't like. The general premise of almost all nutrition plans for a disease such as mine is that certain foods trigger inflammation and other foods don't. This is all well and good in principle, but they tend to follow a one-size-fits-all approach, and if nothing else, one thing I do know is that different things work for different people.

So, how am I going to fill a whole chapter of a book with any useful information, having just alluded to the fact that my requirements are specifically mine and these may or may not apply to you?

The best advice I can begin with is that you are the only person who can work out what you should be eating and what you should not be eating. This is no easy goal to achieve though. You are bombarded with food marketing all day, every day. This can be from manufacturers selling their products, retailers selling their stocks, experts selling their specialist knowledge, or people in general passing along whatever pieces of information they have acquired. Then, there is also the financial impact of dietary choices to factor in. If you are going to diverge from the standard choices on offer, you are going to find it suddenly becomes more expensive.

I have arrived at something very specific for myself, and I

do think it might have some significant value if you are in any kind of similar situation, but there again, maybe it won't. So rather than just telling you what I found, I'll explain a bit about the process I went through to arrive there. This is probably the more useful part of what I've got to say about food and nutrition, as opposed to actual meal plans.

I spent a long time with some very serious disease, and for much of that time, I couldn't make head nor tail of what was helping me and what was making me worse. I had no clue. Medication kept me alive when I was ill, but that same medication made it even more of an impossibility to work out what I should be eating.

The first food choice I made, long before I stopped taking medicines, was to switch to organic wherever I could. This wasn't, and still isn't, always possible, due to availability and price, but I still do try to have as much organic food as I can. Another thing I did many years ago was to fit a filtration system to my house water supply, as I had a suspicion that the chemicals added to mains tap water to clean it of bugs and parasites were probably not too beneficial otherwise. I've maintained these filters ever since. My thinking behind the organic food and filtered water was, and still is, there's no way artificial chemicals can be good for you. The best-case scenario is that they are not detrimental to health, but that is the best you can argue. So, organic food and chemical-free water aside, what else do I factor into my eating equations?

First of all, I'm in a bit of a different situation from that of most other people. This is because I've had rather a lot of my digestive system removed over the years, and have had active disease right through what remains, at various times. This means my basic aim is towards nutrient-dense foods that don't require too much processing internally, specifically ones that don't contain much that is not a direct nutrient. Organic helps towards this aim, along with my filtered water.

In terms of what counts as nutrients, most people know the basic groupings of foodstuffs, which are protein, fat, and carbohydrates. Vitamins and minerals are contained in varying proportions within these major groups. I don't consider fibre to be a nutrient as such, because it is not absorbed by the body. Its function is mostly to maintain the transit of other fibre.

We need protein, which gets broken down into amino acids by the digestive process. The amino acids are absorbed into the bloodstream and transported to cells to act as building blocks for our protein requirements.

Protein-rich foods include meat, eggs, and dairy products. I'm not going to go into ethics or anything here, just the raw content of different foodstuffs, and this being the case, these are the best sources of protein, full stop. With the possible exception of dairy products, they are also the easiest to digest, at least if your digestive system is producing acid. They contain lots of fat, which is good, and also lots of vitamins and minerals.

Fat is essential to life. There is a bit of an ideological dislike of fats in modern society, but without fat, we could not survive. It is essential for the creation and maintenance of cell membranes, among other things.

Of particular note, a thing called the myelin sheath wraps and protects the nerves, and fat is required for that, along with protein. The function of the myelin sheath is to insulate nerves from external electrical signals, as well as speed up the transmission of electricity through the nervous system. This is something you most definitely want to keep intact. It makes your brain and your entire nervous system work, which in turn makes all the other parts of you work.

Carbohydrate isn't as essential as protein and fat. It is broken down into simple sugars by the digestive process, and these sugars are absorbed into the blood. If you don't eat carbohydrates, your body can synthesise its glucose. Simple sugar in food is absorbed quickly since it doesn't need to be broken down much, and this is why eating lots of sugar in one go gives you a sugar high followed by a sugar low. It all goes in at once and this stimulates the body to produce insulin to transport it away from the blood and into the cells. Once all the additional sugar is used up there is still excess insulin, and this continues to pull sugar out of the blood, leading to low blood sugar situations.

Complex carbohydrates are described as slow release because it takes time for the digestive system to break them down into glucose, so the theory is that only small amounts get absorbed at any one time. That is the theory at least. I can draw on my personal experience of eating meals of complex carbohydrates, getting a sugar rush after a couple of hours, and then suffering a dip soon after. My thinking here is that my digestive process will sometimes make all of the carbohydrates into sugar at the same time, leading to a delayed reaction, but a sugar spike followed by a dip all the same.

All foods contain trace amounts of the vitamins and minerals we need. A decent rock salt contains many more minerals than table salt, which is just sodium chloride. Fruit and vegetables are arguably higher in vitamins than any other food, hence the five-a-day messaging about eating fruit and veg as part of a healthy diet. Plant-based food also contains a lot of fibre, something that is considered a good thing. Maybe not so beneficial in my kind of situation, however.

I could write a whole lot more about nutrients and still get nowhere in terms of explaining the process I have adopted for my particular problems. In basic terms, you need protein, you need fat, you need vitamins, minerals, and to a lesser extent, you could say you need carbohydrates. Although it might be better to say carbohydrates can be enjoyed. Many years of very in-depth research, by people other than myself I should add, concerning all the intricacies of dietary choices has gotten nowhere in terms of explaining Crohn's, so my thinking is that if all the acquired knowledge hasn't helped get to the bottom of the disease, then this isn't the route to such a discovery. The medical establishment also seems to think the same thing, because it can't identify any part of food as being a direct cause. All the professionals can do is repeat popular mantras, namely that sugar, salt, fat, and the like are bad for you.

So rather than looking at the microscopic details of the intricacies of nutrition, I started looking elsewhere.

Many people have tried to come up with some form of definitive advice or set of guidelines, not just for people like me, but for everyone, whatever their background. The result of all this endeavour is many proofs about various aspects of food, but often these proofs will directly contradict another proof that had just as much diligence applied to it. You can find an expert who will state that a specific food is good for you, and then you can find another expert telling you the same one is bad for you. Not much of the advice I have read seems to have come to the conclusions I have, and I think this is because of the mechanistic thinking installed and instilled into scientific minds. This leads to something best described as a quantitative approach, by which I mean quantities of specific elements of foods become the focus of the research.

When approaching the subject from this perspective there seems to be a tendency to disregard the quality of the foods that the supposed ideal quantities are being derived from, and this means there is a rather large blind spot covering a great deal of research. The quality of food, as well as referring to proportions of nutrients, also must include things like production and preparation methods to form a complete picture, as every stage in the process potentially adds to, or takes something away from, whatever ends up on your plate. The nature of science is to isolate whatever is being studied, and with food, this means isolation to the study of the finished product, followed by isolation of the finished product into the identifiable nutrients contained within it. As with my explanation in an earlier chapter when I was discussing ulceration and inflammation, the process of isolation means that it is entirely possible to disregard the very things that might point to the source of a problem, namely whatever is in there that is not being looked for.

It should also be noted that the digestive system itself is often viewed as a constant in terms of nutrition when nothing could be further from the truth.

My main focus has been to find a method I can apply to myself, one that will remain true in all circumstances. So if you find some of my reasoning in what is to follow to be not what you would expect from a typical scientific approach, all I am looking for is a system I can use to inform my actions. Think back to my explanation of logical and physical models in computer programming. It isn't necessary to have an intricate understanding of things to build an effective model, as long as you have a precise idea of how those things exert influence at the level your model exists at. The choices I make regarding nutrition get to play out in real life when I apply them, and this has provided a very effective way of ensuring the steps I take are accurate.

For most of my life, I've been told saturated fat is bad, and unsaturated fats are good, but that all fat intake should be kept to a minimum. I've been told that saturated fats make you have heart attacks and also make you overweight and unhealthy. However, I also remember how, in the 1970s, everything was cooked in lard or beef dripping (which was reused over and over again until there were too many bits and pieces in the pan, at which point it was either replaced or had the bits sieved out). People generally seemed healthy enough back then. Furthermore, I remember how this all changed in the 1980s when 'healthy' vegetable oils replaced those artery-clogging animal fats. My own experience of fats is that the ones promoted as healthy are anything but, and I've possibly got some explaining to do before you will believe me on this front.

I'm not about to go too far into the science of fats, because that is a very extensive and expansive subject, and it ultimately tells me nothing about how they affect me personally. Instead, I'm going to look at how different fats and oils are made, and see what conclusions this can lead to...

Olive oil is made by squashing and squeezing olives and collecting the oil that comes out of them. So that is probably OK in terms of being fit for consumption, as there is nothing else in there but the oil that comes out of the olives. The longevity of people living around the Mediterranean also might provide some additional evidence that it is good, as people from that region tend to live longer than people in other places. However, their longevity might also simply be because they live in a nice warm climate so don't have the same kinds of struggles as people in more northerly places.

For coconut oil, there are several production methods, involving heating, pressing, or soaking the flesh of the coconut, but essentially the oil just comes straight out of the flesh. So that would seem to be fairly natural also. As with places where olive oil comes from, the people in areas that use coconut oil tend to live longer than average. As with the Mediterranean though, these are hot places, so, playing Devil's advocate, maybe the climate is something of a contributing factor.

Now animal fats. The most common of these are lard from pigs, then beef dripping or tallow from cows. These are produced by heating the fatty bits of the animal (it is dead at this point by the way), collecting the fat that comes out as a liquid, and then allowing it to set. So, notwithstanding your views regarding the ethics and morality of doing such a thing, these fats are pretty much as they exist inside the animal. Animals need fat to survive for the same reasons we do, and they need the same kind of fat that we do, so putting the issues of dead animals aside, the fat rendered from them is the exact kind of fat we need in our bodies.

I used to joke that if saturated fat was so bad then how come pigs are full of it? I didn't know much about foods at the time but had an inkling this must have illustrated that saturated fat wasn't as bad as it was made out to be. I usually got told to shut up whenever I did say this though.

I will also point out that I know fats are broken down into smaller pieces during digestion, and then reassembled once absorbed into the body, so the fat you eat isn't the fat you end up with inside of you, and your body will also make additional fat out of carbohydrates. However, if you eat fats of the kind your body requires, those broken-down pieces will have an easier path towards reassembly back into a similar kind of fat that was broken down in the first place.

Butter next, and this is made by agitating high-fat cream until the buttermilk separates from it, leaving a solid block of butter, which is just the concentrated fat out of the cream. So there's arguably nothing bad there.

Vegetable, or seed oil, includes the likes of rapeseed (or canola) and sunflower. The fats I have looked at up to now have fairly simple methods of extraction, but that is all about to change with vegetable oils.

The most common oil is rapeseed, which was renamed canola in the 1970s when a new strain of the rapeseed plant was developed through selective breeding. The reason why this was necessary was that standard rapeseed oil contains high levels of erucic acid, which is poisonous. So when you read an article telling you how rapeseed oil is one of the oldest oils used in human history, the articles tend to downplay the fact that all it was good for until very recently was lamp oil or lubrication of machinery. The canola plant, or more correctly the canola strain of rapeseed marked the first time when 'food grade' oil could be extracted from the rapeseed plant.

Canola apparently has very low levels of erucic acid, so all is good according to the industry that manufactures the oil, and all is also good according to the regulators that rubber-stamp it as fit for consumption and a pro-health choice. I can't for the life of me find out what the level of erucic acid is in canola oil, but I can rest assured that it is low enough to be considered safe. Now I might argue that none at all is the only safe amount, but there again, what do I know?

I could introduce a line of reasoning into this using cyanide as an example. If you had a food product that contained cyanide (and believe it or not such a thing is probably in your cupboard if you use standard table salt) then you might be justified in having one or two slight concerns about the overall safety of that product. However, the food standards people will assure you that it is perfectly safe because they have done testing and have produced a piece of paper saying it is safe. Yet regardless of this, you might have a nagging concern because you know there is no safe level of cyanide, and you would be right to have that concern. But there it is, in your table salt, Sodium Hexacyanoferrate.

A quote from a food additives website is, "Many salts of cyanide are dangerous, but the cyanide in food grade ferro-cyanides is non-toxic as it is tightly bound to an iron atom and so **does not tend to release free cyanide**."

I've highlighted the end of that quote because this is a very different statement from one saying it does not release cyanide at all. Now, you probably know that salt is linked to heart disease. Along with butter and lard, you've had this message beaten into you for most of your lifetime. It is quite interesting however that the toxicity of cyanide also causes heart problems. Add that to the 'does not tend' part of the statement above and you might then have to rethink your stance on salt. While you are doing this, I'd advise that you switch to rock salt or sea salt with nothing added for anti-caking purposes. Rock salt is probably better because the cleanliness of the sea is a bit of an ongoing issue.

Anyway, back to vegetable oil and erucic acid. Interestingly, erucic acid also causes cardiac problems. As I said just before, I'd say that none at all would be the ideal amount to be ingesting, not just low levels of it. Erucic acid aside, the next thing to do is to look into how dry, hard little seeds are turned into a bottle of oil. It seems the industry doesn't want to go too far into this. There are various processes, the main distinction being between cold-pressed and standard production methods.

The standard method of production involves heating, crushing, cooking, adding solvents, bleaching, deodorising, sometimes partially hydrogenating, then 'removing' the solvents. I'll get to hydrogenation in a minute, but the rest of the process must affect the alleged goodness of the product. A search on the internet gives you some limited information about the manufacturing stages, but in true Soviet style, it directs you to plenty of information about how much is produced each year. Even when you get to production methods, there isn't much information relating to residual contamination, and that provides you with a clue as to the direction I am going in with my musings on food.

Vegetable oils require many production steps to turn the seeds of a plant into a bottle of oil on a supermarket shelf. Each stage of this process brings with it the potential for some amount of contamination to enter into the finished product. By contamination, I mean one or more substances that are not in any way nutritionally beneficial. These might be below any regulatory threshold, and might even be classed as non-toxic and therefore of little consequence, but they remain in the final product, nonetheless.

The cold-pressed side of the rapeseed industry claims that it only presses the seeds and collects the oil, which makes you wonder why the normal production methods use so many chemicals and industrial processes to get the same stuff out of the same raw material, but there you go.

Something you might see as being somewhat anecdotal is my

pet dog providing me with all the proof I need that vegetable oil maybe isn't as good as it is presented as being.

If I get some chicken or something and fry it in lard or beef dripping, then offer it to my dog, in typical dog fashion he will just about bite off a bit of my hand along with the chicken when I offer it to him. If I fry the chicken in vegetable oil and then offer some of this to him, he will sniff at it for a while, then will turn it down.

Dogs will eat almost anything, and my dog is no exception. He will even eat his own shit given the chance, and if I was to spew up upon seeing such a sight, he'd happily proceed to lap up my sick. However, given the offer of some prime chicken smothered in vegetable oil, he does not recognise it as food. That alone is all I need to inform me that vegetable oil is not the best thing in terms of nutrition. Before you jump to the conclusion that dogs are stupid, to which I'll agree that they don't possess the same reasoning capabilities as us (and my dog is admittedly a bit of an idiot, even in dog terms), I'll just point out that the nose of a dog is one of the true wonders of nature.

OK then, next is hydrogenation, and its close cousin, partial hydrogenation. The purpose of hydrogenating vegetable oil is to push it towards being more solid at room temperature. This makes it more appropriate for making things like manufactured cakes and biscuits because you want such items to be stable, solid, and most certainly not seeping and oozing out of the bottom of the packaging on a warm day. Hydrogenated oil also acts as a preservative, thereby increasing shelf life.

Margarine, which surprisingly (to me, at least) has been in existence since the 1800s, only became popular after the Second World War. Originally made from beef tallow, over time it changed to being made from hydrogenated vegetable oil. Fully hydrogenated oils are hard and waxy at room temperature, so are not entirely ideal for use as a spread, or as a baking ingredient. Partially hydrogenated oils are a lot softer, so will spread and mix more easily, just what you want when looking for something that resembles butter. Unfortunately, partially hydrogenated oils contain trans fatty acids, and these are incredibly bad for you. They are more than just linked to heart disease, and as such are being removed from many of the products they used to be in, although interestingly, the heat-based production methods of seed oils are alleged to convert the healthy Omega-3's (one of the major selling points) into trans-fats. Many brands of margarine have now switched over to the use of palm oil, which is probably better unless you begin to ask questions about tropical deforestation.

There is a certain amount of ambiguity surrounding the labelling of ingredients when it comes to hydrogenated oils. An ingredient listed as 'hydrogenated oil' is technically correct, whether this refers to full or partial hydrogenation. Also, the hydrogenation process typically involves a nickel catalyst and high temperatures. As with the production of seed oils, this is an industrial process, and as such, I reserve the right to raise the possibility of unspecified contamination, however insignificant, in the end product. Additionally, when making something into a thing that resembles something else, butter in the case of spreads, more ingredients may well be added, things like emulsifiers, dyes, and flavour enhancements.

So, regardless of all the official information regarding fats and oils, I have chosen to go with the ones I have been told are bad for my health. Specifically, I get less indigestion if I stick with lard, dripping, butter, coconut, and olive oils. As an example, I can eat a big plate of bacon and eggs fried in lots of lard and suffer no ill effects whatsoever. If I eat the same bacon and eggs (meaning equivalent, not the very same bacon and eggs) fried in vegetable oil, I end up with some degree of indigestion.

What if it wasn't the actual food causing problems, whatever that food may be, but the quantity of additional, often unspecified stuff in that food? Notwithstanding the presence of erucic acid at some level in canola or rapeseed oil, and the potential for trans fats in hydrogenated oils, the manufacturing processes provide plenty of scope for additional bits and pieces to hop aboard for the ride to your stomach. Animal fats and oils like coconut and olive don't, at least not to such an extent.

Another thing you will struggle enormously to not have heard about is cholesterol. There was, until very recently, an association between saturated fat intake, high cholesterol, and negative health outcomes. Cholesterol is not a fat as such, in the way that lard and butter are. It belongs to a group of chemicals known as sterols, which are a subgroup of another group called lipids. Fats are also a subgroup of lipids, hence the popular confusion that cholesterol is the same general thing as fat, but it is not. It is the starting point for the body's production of steroids, and these are essential to bodily processes. Most of the cholesterol found in the body is manufactured by the body, rather than being the direct result of dietary input. However, it must be remembered that at some level, everything in the body is the result of something that was eaten at some point, so saying something is not directly linked to food would be better framed in terms of the number of steps removed from the food or foods it started as.

As I said near the start of this chapter, I am neither claiming nor aiming to be an expert in the intricacies of food or internal bodily processes, so I'm not about to start digging much deeper. However, the production of and existence of cholesterol in the body is way more complicated than simply being a negative consequence of eating lard, and even mainstream science is beginning to move towards such a position these days.

I have read several arguments relating to cholesterol that adopt a similar stance to my position regarding digestive health and bacteria, in that they claim high cholesterol is a response to an underlying problem, rather than the cause of that problem. While this does resonate with my general perspective on things, I am not in any position to state categorically that it is the case, or that it is not. However, it remains a point of interest for me.

So, getting back to things found directly in food, I've mentioned the anti-caking agents in table salt, but there are lots of other anti-caking agents in all kinds of ingredients. Aside from the ferrocyanides, aluminium also features heavily in the world of anti-caking agents. I don't remember ever learning that aluminium was good. Silicates are also well represented. I don't have any direct information regarding health benefits or otherwise, but silicate means sand, and you probably don't need to be told not to eat sand. Powdered Cellulose is also used for such purposes, meaning ground-up sawdust or wood pulp. Talc is even listed as an anti-caking agent, and talc has made headlines related to asbestos. All of these kinds of chemicals find their way into various foods and have been doing so for many years.

With meat, eggs, and dairy, organic produce has the least potential to contain any chemical residue. While there are such residues in the air and water now, meaning organic food will contain some level of it, this will still be much lower than the levels in non-organic food, where the chemicals are directly added to it. There is no argument for these kinds of residues being in any way good for you. The only possible position in support of them is that the amounts found in foods are below any agreed toxicity threshold. I don't want to go too much into corporate and government politics here, but there is a great deal of common ground between the worlds of government, big business, and safety regulation.

The people who decide what is safe and what is not are tasked with doing so within the framework of maintaining a functioning economy that can consistently provide the basic resources for a whole population. In contrast, the only way to produce food of the specific quality I am looking for is to follow the best possible practices during production, meaning welfare, environmental, and production considerations are a necessary part of the process, rather than a minimum set of rules imposed by some government agency.

Looking into the more extreme side of dietary choices, some people eat nothing other than meat and eggs, and then other people eat nothing other than meat, eggs, and dairy. There are even people who eat nothing but meat, and some of them even prefer raw meat (which definitely seems a step too far, if you ask me). Such people claim that following such a strict diet will eliminate all inflammation. While I'm not going to refute such claims, I couldn't stick to such a limited diet, and even if I could, I think I would struggle to find the money to do so. So while a large proportion of what I eat is meat, eggs, and to a lesser extent, dairy, I would find it too restrictive if that was all I ate.

After fats and proteins, the other major food group is carbohydrates, and this is where things get a little bit more complicated. Carbohydrate refers to any organic compound containing carbon, hydrogen, and oxygen. It doesn't refer to something that is automatically digestible. Sugars and starches are carbohydrates, and these can be digested. Various types of fibre are also carbohydrates and are not digestible. I already gave you my basic opinion regarding simple sugar in my chapter looking at the Elemental Diet. Since I am discussing food here, I'll state my position again.

Sugar is one of the few things in existence where the mainstream of society is in agreement with the outliers of society, by which I mean the alternative or holistic health industry. No matter where someone places themselves on the spectrum of health advice, the chances are they will hold the view that sugar is very, very bad for you. Maybe it is if you eat too much, although I would place this into a category of over-indulgence rather than one of outright toxicity.

It doesn't seem to affect me too much in terms of negative consequences unless I apply the full bag of it in one go method. Reasonable amounts of sugar don't increase my inflammation, although I will admit that defining what reasonable means is kind of like defining how long a piece of string is.

Some of the more extreme positions people take regarding sugar seem to suggest that it is directly toxic to your body, but I simply can't see how something that your body utilises for energy is also a direct toxin. Yes, too much can certainly be a bad thing for reasons more related to putting stress on how your body processes it, but classifying it as a toxin in and of itself seems a bit of a stretch.

Artificial sweeteners are a different matter entirely though. They do not break down into anything useful, and as such cannot be beneficial to your body. If they get through the barrier of your digestive system and into your blood, then your body is tasked with eliminating them.

My general position on simple sugars is that they are far preferable to artificial sweeteners. Almost all artificial sweeteners have some sort of a link to inflammatory disease hidden somewhere in the research on them. This even includes Stevia, which is marketed as a safe, natural alternative. My direct observations regarding sweeteners include them being the direct cause of indigestion, or failing that, my inflammation has tended to be worse when not specifically avoiding them, whereas I can't find a similar link between good old-fashioned sugar and negative consequences.

I tend to buy unrefined cane sugar for my needs. Unrefined sugar has a brownish colour, which is due to molasses that hasn't been removed by refining processes. Molasses has a few more nutrients in it than basic white sugar.

Starches are next on my list. A starch is a complex carbohydrate consisting of a long chain of glucose molecules. These are in things like rice, flour, and potatoes. They are broken down into glucose in the digestive system, and this is absorbed into the bloodstream, where it provides energy to the body. I'm fine with rice, have never got on too well with potatoes, and for the past year or so have avoided all wheat products. I'm OK with oats and maize though (maize is very often and unhelpfully known as corn, but oats, barley, rye, and wheat are also types of corn). Carbohydrate-rich foods also tend to contain more than just the sugars and starches that we can digest, and this is where the complexity sets in.

I avoid wheat and barley because of the gluten in them, and gluten, which is a protein, has a long history of causing problems in enough people for it to be seen as significant. I never noticed any problem with it until I stopped taking all my medication. As soon as I was free from omeprazole, I began to notice that I would begin to experience indigestion, followed by diarrhoea a few hours after eating any foods containing gluten. I honestly don't think it had ever been too much of a problem before I was ill, and the medications I took for many years stopped me from noticing if and when it became an issue.

This was a big problem, to begin with, as just like a vast number of people, wheat formed most of my staple diet. It found its way into almost every meal or snack I was eating, right throughout every single day. It was difficult to identify as a problem since it was in my system constantly, and I therefore had no baseline state to compare with.

Once I realised that wheat, or more specifically gluten, was causing me problems, I struggled to come up with an alternative way of eating. Initially, I gravitated towards meat and eggs only, but couldn't hold my weight just eating those things, so I tried gluten-free alternatives to wheat. This led me to the 'Free From' aisles of the supermarkets. To start with, I seemed to get along fine with gluten-free bread and other snacks. The only difference was that the gluten-free alternatives were incredibly expensive in comparison, and tasted awful. If you remember back to my Elemental Diet chapter, I mentioned that the backlog in the health service worked in my favour. The reason for this was that during this time I had identified gluten as a problem, and by the time I tried the Elemental drinks, I was starting to make some actual headway in terms of discovering what was sustaining my ongoing disease.

One theory surrounding gluten is that since it is a small protein molecule, and is said to be fairly resistant to digestive enzymes, it can find its way through the epithelial layer of the digestive tract and therefore into the bloodstream as a gluten molecule, rather than as digested amino acids. The body doesn't recognise the gluten molecule as being a nutrient but sees it as a foreign particle, meaning it mounts an immune response. Hence inflammation, which if not addressed by avoiding gluten, is potentially going to get worse over time.

Gluten-free foods began to cause the same problems that had led to me removing gluten in the first place. At first glance, this might seem to mean gluten was never the problem, but I went in a different direction with my reasoning about what was happening.

I had temporarily solved the problems I was experiencing due to gluten, so rather than just giving up on my experiment, I began to look for something in gluten-free foods that could cause the same problems. I found it in the form of xanthan gum.

Xanthan gum is a polysaccharide, so in the same basic chemical family as monosaccharides, or simple sugars, but a bigger molecule. It is water soluble and cannot be broken down into simple sugars by the digestive system, giving rise to it being part of a category of substances known as soluble fibres, also known as prebiotics. So it will dissolve in water but cannot be turned into a nutrient for the body. When dissolved in water it becomes a gloopy, gelatinous mixture, kind of like wallpaper paste.

This turned out to be the final piece of the jigsaw I had been trying to put together for most of my life. If gluten was getting to places it had no business being, and my body was responding by seeing it as an attack, and then if xanthan gum was causing the very same issues, the only logical conclusion was that it was also getting to the same inappropriate places and my body was mounting the same response as it had been with gluten (*). From that point everything made sense.

*Just for context, I don't know if things like gluten and soluble fibre are actually getting through my overstretched defences and into my blood, or if they are just interfering with what I have in the way of mucous membrane, the first barrier to stuff getting where it shouldn't. For my purposes though, this distinction does not matter. I can perceive it as things getting to my blood, or I can perceive it as some getting that far and other stuff just affecting or displacing my mucous, or can even perceive it as everything putting additional stress on the mucous alone. Whatever the actual case, the result is the same, namely irritation, followed by ulceration and inflammation.

From the onset of my Crohn's Disease many years ago, I always had varying amounts of difficulty with fruits and vegetables. I haven't mentioned these foods very much up to now, and this is because I could never make much sense of what to do about them. We get bombarded with information regarding the benefits of fruit and veg, with messages telling us they are the route to good health. All other foods are presented as being less than ideal for one reason or another, but you will struggle to hear a bad word about fruits and vegetables. My experience with them is somewhat different to the endless benefits I am told about, with my own 'beneficial' outcomes ranging from indigestion to fullness and bloating, right through to severe pains and emergency admission to hospital when the skin or seeds caused blockages in my digestive system.

Not being able to do the thing you are told you must do to be healthy is something of a trauma-inducing situation, but as with earlier in the book, I'm still trying my hardest not to moan about anything, so I won't tell you any more about how bad it made me feel when I simply couldn't eat any fruit or veg, even though I have just managed to slip in this little comment about just that.

The immediately obvious issue is the visible indigestible parts of fruits and vegetables, better explained as their fibrous content. Roughage-type fibre is easy to explain in terms of the state of my digestion. I had a propensity for developing strictures, so the big bits and pieces would get stuck if I hadn't chewed them up enough. At times when I didn't have strictures, such as after surgery to remove them, fruit and veg would often still cause me quite a bit of indigestion, and I could not understand why. Even so, I did try my hardest to eat them, mainly because I was indoctrinated to believe that I needed the goodness contained in them.

When I finally linked why gluten and xanthan gum gave me the same basic issues, namely that they were getting to places where they caused irritation, the pieces of the jigsaw relating to fruits and vegetables also fell into place, as they contain lots of indigestible parts, not just the big bits of skin and the seeds, but also various soluble fibres. I began to wonder if these soluble fibres were doing much the same thing, namely getting through my defences instead of remaining contained in my digestive system, and then causing the irritation, ulceration, and inflammation that were diagnosed as my ongoing disease. If I take soluble fibre supplements, or prebiotics as they are more commonly marketed, then I get the very same indigestion that results from foods containing gluten or xanthan gum.

So, after 36 years I finally had a working model to go with. This doesn't explain why I got like this in the first place, but it does explain why my problems persisted for so long. My thinking was that I was constantly ingesting more of the very things required to perpetuate my issues.

Once I arrived at this line of reasoning, I started looking for other things that might be having the same effect, or that might have had the same effect in the past. Playing it safe, I decided to remove as many artificial ingredients as possible from my diet, with the thought that any or all such things might not be recognised by my blood as being a nutrient or as being harmless. I had already removed the likes of excess residual contaminants by going organic, maltodextrin for reasons to do with the mucous membrane of the digestive tract and artificial sweeteners for various similar reasons. If I applied my new line of reasoning to most, if not all of these, it held.

Of particular note is microcrystalline cellulose. This is a bulking agent used in all sorts of foods, and particularly as a base for tablet-based medicines and nutritional supplements. It is also used as an anti-caking agent but is called powdered cellulose for such purposes. Microcrystalline cellulose is ground-down sawdust. Termites can digest wood. Cows are also able to, to an extent, but they have very specialised stomachs to work with. Humans don't have this capacity. Microcrystalline cellulose, as the name suggests, consists of very small particles, only visible through a microscope. If my ongoing problems were the result of small particles getting through the defences in my gut and to places they had no business getting to, then small particles such as ground-down sawdust could also be doing the same thing.

To put all of this in the simplest terms, I now think of anything indigestible or artificial as being something like grit or dust. I'm not too concerned about what it specifically is, but if it is there in whatever food might be containing it, it is going to get to places it shouldn't and cause problems.

I am not going to advocate for any rigid diet plan, something I think is detrimental to the nature of life, which is a state of constant flux. I will also state my opinion that the condition of a person's digestive system is as unique as their fingerprint, so a one-size-fits-all approach is never going to work. But for me, the problem seems to be all of the little bits of stuff that are not nutrients.

A quick summary of what I do eat is mostly meat and eggs, cooked in saturated fat when required. I get through a bit of milk and cream, sticking with lactose-free options most of the time, to give my digestive system less work to do. All of this is organic where possible, free range / outdoor bred where not, and cheaper, lower quality versions when circumstances make that the only option (the most common circumstance leading to this is the amount of money in my pocket).

I bake a few 'nice' things from scratch, as I do have a sweet tooth. So this includes biscuits and one or two bakery items, but options are limited here since I use either cornflour or gluten-free flour, which are nothing like wheat flour (gluten-free waffles work fine and muffins are just about edible, but bread of any kind is off my menu). Other ingredients in my baked items are sugar (in the form of actual sugar, maple syrup, or honey), eggs, milk, butter, oats, and coconut. I use either well-filtered water or spring water. I do add various spices to meals, but never in the form of off-the-shelf sauces. I also get through lots of Himalayan rock salt.

I avoid anything that has the potential to contain small indigestible bits that might aggravate whatever damage is already present. My list of things to avoid is soluble fibre (or prebiotics), all artificial sweeteners, gluten, all bulking agents, fillers, thickeners, and emulsifiers, lactose (to an extent), microcrystalline cellulose (sawdust), anything with a name starting with *mono*, or *poly*, or *di*, or *tri*, and anything else that sounds as if it came out of a laboratory or factory. I also steer well clear of vegetable oils, whether hydrogenated or not.

The avoidance of soluble fibre means I avoid almost all fruit and veg. An anomaly is sweetcorn, which seems fine, even though it contains a lot of fibre. However, the fibre is mostly insoluble, and it doesn't present me with any problems at the moment.

I also don't eat nuts, but since this is something I've never really done, I can't say whether they are specifically problematic for me or not. I have an inkling the chunks they tend to chew up into would cause problems, but I'm not in any hurry to test this.

Since I have a sweet tooth, I will eat sweets (candy if you are American), but stick to things that are made with gelatine rather than pectin (a soluble fibre from fruit), ones with real sugar rather than artificial sweeteners, and ones with natural rather than artificial flavours.

I drink some coffee each day, made with sugar and milk. I also like fizzy pop (soda if you are American). Unfortunately, the UK government is waging an ongoing war against sugar, and has succeeded in destroying the soft drinks industry, by which I mean there are very few drinks left that aren't sweetened with some chemical as opposed to sugar. As such I have been forced to make my fizzy pop, using sparkling spring water, and high-end cordial (because the sugar tax has also ruined most of the available squash), but I add copious amounts of sodium ascorbate to the drinks I make, meaning I get up to ten grams of vitamin C each day through this route, or at least on the days I remember to make it. So on the days I do remember, I get through considerable amounts of vitamin C.

I don't take any other vitamins or supplements, apart from the occasional high-dose course of vitamin D3, usually during winter months. This is the expensive version of vitamin D tablets, ones that do not contain any bulking agents. As I write this, I did buy some for this autumn, but have completely forgotten to take them up to now, and I am currently looking at snow on the ground out of my window.

Effectively, this means the vast majority of food products in a grocery store are on my avoid list, which might sound very limiting, but I am stable for the first time in almost forty years. My results are looking better each time I have blood tests. My weight is holding steady. I get to the end of each day without any indigestion. My doctors can't understand why.

I'll also point out, that the brief description of the kinds of foods I do eat is probably enough to give a variety of experts more than a few palpitations. In general, it is everything I've always been told not to eat. All of this could be construed as yet another solution causing the problem. The solution here is related to overcoming the problems of poor health and lower longevity, and in terms of what is considered the best advice, almost all official sources are singing from the same songbook. This includes the medical industry, the government, the health and wellness industry, and the mainstream media. I can't speak for anyone else, but for me, the endless advice about good, healthy nutrition seems to have perpetuated many years of just the opposite.

The one place where I do apply diligence is with the little

indigestible bits, things that go unnoticed by almost every authority on the subject, and nobody has ever advised me to do that.

9

My Unified Theory Of My Disease

Right back at the start of this book, I said I could fit what I needed to say about my version of Crohn's into a pamphlet, or maybe even onto a single sheet of paper. I can go one better than this if I narrow it down to how I resolved the disease, and fit it into a single sentence...

For me, my ongoing inflammation was the result of indigestible bits in food, specifically molecules or pieces of whatever else that are not nutrients, but are small enough to make it through the barrier of my digestive system and to places where they cause damage or just trigger an immune response, meaning the solution is to not eat those indigestible bits.

So there you go, it is as easy as that. Maybe or maybe not for you, but it most certainly is for me. The way to resolve my issues has simply been to not ingest the things that were causing the issues. It makes for a rather odd diet, but this is far more beneficial than sticking with regular food and having to keep my inflammation.

It doesn't require a medical degree to understand this and is not the result of any expensive and complex research. The self-perpetuating nature of my disease was just a response to environmental factors, and the solution was to limit my exposure to those factors.

I need to clarify what I have just said, mainly to prevent people of science from shooting my findings down. I am not looking for the specific chemical or biological pathways behind what I am describing. My approach would be better described as a meta-analysis, one where common elements are the focus of my attention. This is what is important, as it allows me to find ways of navigating around my problems. I am not interested in the microscopic details of things like what molecule is affecting which group of cells, or what is specifically triggering certain responses inside of me.

I have aimed to construct the simplest possible working model to meet my needs. As long as there are no observable situations where this fails, then it is still entirely valid to use it. Many doctors or other scientists will claim otherwise, but it is worth remembering that all of their highly intricate knowledge has completely failed to help me in any way whatsoever. So, if I say it is as simple as things getting through my defences and into places it shouldn't, then I take action based on this assumption, and that action has the desired result, then my model is valid, whether or not it is entirely accurate down to the finest of details.

The root of the problem as I see it, or at least the root of the expression of the problem, is related to the protective layer of mucous in my digestive system. There may well be several reasons why mine was not up to the task of doing what it should have been doing, namely protecting my actual cells.

You might have heard that up to 90% of the immune system is in the digestive system, but you might not have been given much context as to what this means. I know it is something I have heard many times, without any further explanation about it. As far as I can tell though, it seems to be alluding to the fact that a good layer of protection is going to stop potentially damaging particles from getting through it, as opposed to being part of some intelligent and intricate network of immune circuitry. If, like me, you don't have that layer of protection, then the only solution is to make sure offending particles don't pass your lips.

Something I mentioned early on was the idea that to develop a serious illness, several different influencing factors must be present. So while my solution to my disease is to apply simple rules regarding food, the reasons why it developed in the first place are rather more difficult to pin down. The rest of this chapter is a discussion of these influences, which are not particularly relevant to the very straightforward actions I have adopted. The things I am going to mention here are things that I perhaps could have addressed back in the mists of time, and if I had done so I'd potentially not have gone on to develop problems. However, the time to do so has passed, so while they may have helped nudge me towards the situation I found myself in, there's nothing I can do to change them now.

I started the first chapter by saying there is never an absolute starting point, which means the event that triggered my disease, namely my BCG vaccine, cannot be seen as the whole reason behind it, or even the main reason for that matter. It is not entirely possible to define everything that led to an injection causing such an outcome in me, but not in the vast majority of people who also received the same injection. However, I will say that mass medication can never work as intended, because to do so would require everyone to be an exact clone of everyone else.

There is a psychological backdrop to all physical illness. The medical position regarding this is a bit different to how I see it. While medicine does acknowledge psychological processes relating to disease, it sees them in terms of the effects on the mind being a result of the disease. I don't see anything wrong with this, as your physical condition does have a huge impact on your mental processes. Lack of energy, pain, and constantly feeling rotten affect your thinking tremendously.

Where I will go a bit further than standard science, is in saying that your mental landscape can potentially play a huge role in the kind of disease you will go on to develop. Medicine doesn't go much further than attributing certain diseases to lifestyle choices, but I have something of an inkling that things go a bit deeper.

I've previously mentioned how the disease I got to experience mirrored my state of mind, and gave me a physical manifestation of my lack of confidence, specifically putting it on display for all to see, regardless of what I tried to do to hide my shortcomings. The obvious next question is why.

Even the most committed materialist must surely admit that the mind and the body maintain feedback loops to one another. At the most basic level, the condition of the body informs the mind as to what the body is capable of, and the mind then selects behaviours it believes the body can manage. These actions then either confirm, or dispel, the original belief in the mind, and this informs future choices. Behavioural loops develop when choices and actions repeatedly feed the same results back. This is somewhere near the core of why we develop distinct personalities, both for the positive and the negative aspects of our characters.

The nature of a loop, being circular, means it can be very

difficult to define how, where, and why it started. So, while a pattern of behaviour could express itself mostly in terms of its physical attributes, or alternately by a psychological perspective, the origin of any such pattern could just as easily reside in the mind or the body.

There is, I think, a very strong case for the root of disease, certainly for chronic, but possibly all diseases, to reside in the mind. At the same time though, mental roots may develop as a result of some physical trauma. I am describing circles within circles here, something I think presents a fairly strong case for the actual origin of any disease being rather difficult to find. Also, the same disease could have very different starting points for everyone affected by it.

Once you have one or other type of disease, it is also logical to assume this then acts as a very powerful feedback loop into whatever processes might have led to it in the first place, as the physical effects will force you into specific behaviours as a coping mechanism, and, if you dig deep enough, these will possibly align with the mental landscape you started with.

Since the mind informs the body and the body informs the mind, you are then going to struggle with various impossible situations if you try reversing that cycle. Getting out of a loop is not easy, and anyone who tells you otherwise isn't helping. It isn't as simple as doing some exercise and going to bed early, or following some self-help plan, mainly because whatever led you to disease will mean you are not going to be capable of actually keeping up with whatever regime would help. It is more a case of small steps to lessen the wrong thoughts and actions, replacing them with more appropriate things as you go, and a gradual chipping away of anything that is holding you in your current situation.

I'm not going to go too much further into this dynamic, mainly because I am not knowledgeable enough concerning the psychology and physiology of it all. However, if you make the right decisions concerning your physical well-being, your mental situation will follow along, to an extent. The same is true from the other direction. If you identify the problems in your mind, and then take steps to think in a better way, your physical condition will follow along. Doing either or both of these will take a long time to show results though. You can't buy this process from anyone else. It is something you have to do yourself, as everyone has unique problems.

So, returning to where I started, why might a vaccine have triggered a near-endless cycle of inflammatory disease in my particular case?

I think the only answer to this is that I was already very close to developing that disease and the added pressure of eliminating the vaccine ingredients from my body was the straw that broke the camel's back. Please understand though, I'm not giving a free pass to the vaccine here. There are two sides to it, and the fact remains it did initiate a whole set of problems in me, problems that might never have developed otherwise. However, I do think I was already in something of a perilous position, making that vaccine the last thing needed to tip my health into a very negative cycle.

I'm going to explain a few bits and pieces from some of my earliest memories through to when I first became ill. None of this is particularly extreme by any standards, so most of it should just be classed as the normal experiences of childhood. However, I do think that for me, it was enough to start up the loops in my mind and body that led to my subsequent illness. The point here is that it doesn't necessarily have to be the result of any major traumas, but can just as easily be due to a series of fairly regular situations, perhaps with some confluence related to the timing of them.

I had problems with food from an early age. It wasn't an attention thing, or at least I don't think it was. I remember certain foods triggering a vomiting response as soon as I started to chew them, without any conscious contribution to that response. It was more along the lines of putting food in my mouth, biting down on it, and then spewing up immediately. There was no time for thinking about it. I still have this, but avoid anything that might make it happen. The most common type of food that does it is root vegetables cooked to a point where they are soft, particularly if they are also watery. This includes potato, so for a long time I haven't tried to eat boiled potato or home-made chips (French Fries if you are not British, but in the very British style of thick cut and deep fried to a soft, mushy, greasy consistency). It also includes things like turnips, carrots, boiled beetroot, and any other vegetable that disintegrates between my teeth when chewed. So vegetable stews have been off my menu forever. I have no real idea what led to this response in me, and whether it was always there or whether I learned it at some point. Mashed potato has the same effect unless I mix a bit of meat into each mouthful. Rice pudding does the same. So does lumpy soup. Just the smell of over-boiled cabbage has the same effect – that doesn't even need to get into my mouth.

I do remember being forced to eat prunes in pink custard once at my first school, spewing it back into the bowl because of the lumps in the custard, and then being dragged out of my seat to receive a shaking(*) from the dinner lady. Something as simple as this might have been some sort of starting point for the negative loops that became increasingly intricate as time went on, but it might equally have had nothing to do with them. However, I do vaguely remember that my eating became more of an issue around this time. There again, maybe the fact that my eating was becoming a problem was what led to the school pudding situation.

Shaking must have been in fashion as a great way of teaching children in the late 1970s in primary schools in the UK. If not common to all schools, it was a way to control children in the school I went to. If you did something deemed as wrong, you would get hauled out of your seat, held firmly by the shoulders, and then violently shaken.

Anyway, I developed some rather complex eating requirements. I knew I was making things difficult on myself, even then, but since I had no real idea of why it was happening, it continued. The list of things that would make me sick up the contents of my stomach kept growing.

In terms of how adults perceive this, a lot of children go through periods of similar behaviour around food. This is most often viewed as the child seeking attention or trying to assert power, and in many cases it probably is. Away from home, meaning places like school, my eating problems were generally classified this way, so, to the adults, it looked as if I was just trying it on – seeing if I could get one over on them. I was unable to explain the heavy feeling in my stomach or the fact that some foods would make me spew up before I could swallow them. My body was trying to tell me not to eat certain things, but the people looking after me were telling me I had to eat them, so I struggled on with them.

I know something in all of this is somewhere near the origins of my disease, but I don't know what started my eating problems, whether it was some purely physical signs beginning to play out, or whether it was something in my mind that I projected onto my food habits. Perhaps this will serve to illustrate how hard it can be to identify what initiates an ongoing issue, but my obvious issues with food are one of the roots of my problems.

I could take it back to a vaccine my mother received when she was pregnant with me. This was the RhoGAM vaccine, released in 1968, and given to Rhesus-negative mothers carrying babies with Rhesus-positive fathers, the idea behind it being to stop the mother from developing antibodies to the baby she was carrying, in case the baby turned out to have positive blood. The theory behind it was that if the mother did develop those antibodies, she would pass them to the foetus, and it would then attack its blood. I have no idea if this is an actual thing or not, but the manufacturer of the vaccine is obviously going to say it is, and will no doubt have plenty of scientific evidence to support their claim. Anyway, my mother is convinced that injection was what started all of my problems. I can't say one way or the other whether this is the case, as I can't remember this far back.

If you think there is anything in the field of epigenetics, then I can go back another generation. When my father was born, his mother, so my grandmother, developed tuberculosis, meaning she must have been developing it while carrying him. There is a line of reasoning that things like this pass down through generations, manifesting as something else many years later. To me, it seems entirely plausible, but I can't present any evidence to back that up. However, Crohn's and TB were considered expressions of the same sort of thing at one time.

Back to things I can remember, something else that happened around the time I remember eating problems becoming an issue, was an awkward fall where I twisted my leg and ended up with a hernia. This led to a trip to the hospital for surgery to repair it, and perhaps the hernia itself, or the repair, was the cause of some further damage that slowly began festering away.

Another thing I remember from a year or two later was a feeling of a lack of stability. I must point out this has nothing whatsoever to do with my parents or immediate family situation, which was very safe and secure, but more to do with the life I was born into. I grew up on dairy farms, not as a child of the farm owners, but in a farm worker family. By their nature, farms are out in the middle of nowhere, so there is a tendency for people who work on the farm to also live on the farm, and this living arrangement comes in the form of tied houses.

A tied house is a house that is tied to the job, which, for all intents and purposes, is a throwback to medieval serfdom. It gives the landowners a huge amount of power over their workers, as the threat of losing your job brings with it the threat of rapidly becoming homeless. This implied threat means farm owners get much more control over their workers when compared to more regular forms of employment. They also adjust wages down to account for the rental cost of the house, so it isn't even like you can save up to buy your way out.

I know I'm not unique in having grown up in tied houses, but I understood the basic dynamics in play from the age of about seven when we were uprooted because the threat of losing the house became a reality. We ended up on another farm, in another tied house. From that point on I knew about the fragile nature of working-class life, and didn't take to it very well. It helped to feed into my feelings of instability and general lack of confidence. Anyone can have everything taken away at any point, I know this, but there is at least a bit more room to manoeuvre if your living arrangements are not directly tied to your work.

So I developed a perception of precarious living arrangements, and my eating problems continued. I didn't take well to moving to a new school, as all I had known up to then was a village environment, with maybe twenty or thirty children and two or three teachers in the entire school. The new school was a lot bigger and had many more children in attendance. I struggled enormously to fit in but didn't tell my parents, because I also understood the turmoil they had just been through regarding work and housing, and didn't want to further burden them. I learned to pretend everything was good, even though I felt nothing like that.

My problems with eating might have had nothing to do with any of the other circumstances, but they did get worse with each additional situation. I will readily admit that none of this ranks at all on any scale of real traumatic experience. For the most part, I didn't respond well to changes and perceived threats, as opposed to there being any real dangers.

I came up with the idea of escaping this life by writing computer games, something that a handful of people were doing at the time (this was 1982 or thereabouts), so from the age of about 9, I placed a huge amount of pressure on myself to learn game programming. The plan to make my fortune never worked out, but I did get very good at programming computers. Much of my childhood was focused on it, so I would do all of my schoolwork, and then teach myself how to write code. There is an undercurrent of ongoing stress when you do something like this, and maybe that added to my ever-growing issues. It also led me to believe I was going to escape from the harsh realities of working life, so I didn't develop any coping strategies for the real world.

That is the best of what I can dredge up from my early years about how my psychological profile developed towards that of a person with a digestive disease. There are plenty more bits and pieces I can think of, but for the most part, they are more of the same kinds of things. I can frame it all in very simple terms through the use of language, and say that I couldn't digest the circumstances of my life, or perhaps it might be better to say I couldn't stomach them. I do think that simple language constructs can sometimes get straight to the core of whatever is underlying a situation. This is something very easily overlooked in our modern, technological, expert-led, computer-driven age.

There is an aspect of Crohn's that I can certainly apply to my childhood, and I have an inkling it might be fairly common in people with similar illnesses. I might be completely wrong about other people, but if I had to bet money on it, I'd go with it being the case. I remember feelings of never being good enough, not trying hard enough, and not deserving the kinds of things other people took for granted. Rather than this being front and centre stage in my mind, it was more like a little voice, but always there in the background. Having something like this leads to a tendency to compensate via over-achievement. Before becoming ill, my expression of this was my aim towards becoming a world-renowned games programmer, to prove I was good enough, was trying hard enough, and was deserving. When my disease developed, I redirected some of that attention into showing that I could still manage perfectly well. This might, in part at least, explain why Crohn's is not always perceived as the severely debilitating condition that it is, and this being the case, would suggest that many affected people share similar characteristics.

Aside from how my mind developed, it is also worth looking at how the nature of food and farming changed, as this probably also has a great deal of relevance.

One major change was the switch to seed oils from saturated fats. I covered my thoughts on fats and oils in the previous chapter. Just in case you are wondering, a fat is solid and an oil is liquid at room temperature, and just in case you have forgotten what I said earlier, I generally wouldn't touch a seed oil with a barge pole (but if I have to, I will pick sunflower before rapeseed).

Another big change was the increased use of chemicals in farming. This includes things like fertilizers, herbicides, and pesticides, sprayed on growing crops (along with crop varieties specifically designed to withstand such chemicals at levels that will kill anything else), growth hormones, antibiotics, and more pesticides on animals, and things like preservatives and fungicides on harvested crops and feeds. The countryside had been changing for a long time as a result of industrialisation, but when I was young it was changing very rapidly from anything resembling a traditional image of a natural environment into something more like an industrial processing plant. Regardless of how many studies there are to prove how safe all of these chemicals are, there is no way we can continually douse all of our food sources with toxic substances and then expect no negative consequences.

Studies will typically look at each chemical on its own, over a limited time frame, and very often in a tightly controlled environment. Nothing is looking at the effect of them all together, and there is an equal lack of insight into the cumulative effect over a lifetime. At the least, and this is the very least, all those chemicals are going to displace some amount of actual nutrients from the foods they are contained in, so weight for weight, a quantity of food produced with chemical assistance is going to be less nutritious than the same quantity of the same food produced without any chemicals. I'd say it is probably a great deal worse than that, because many of the chemicals used are, by their very nature, designed to kill living things, and any amount of this kind of chemical residue in any particular food is going to continue to kill things. Maybe not an entire living human being, but it cannot be having a beneficial impact on a person's insides.

In addition to the widespread use of chemicals in food production, processed food became much more widespread. There are the obvious kinds of processed food, such as ready meals and snacks, but the ingredients in many basic store cupboard items changed for the worse. Bulking agents allowed for the actual nutrients in a wide range of items to be stretched ever more thinly. To make up for the resulting lack of taste and colour, lots of artificial ingredients were added, to make products that looked, smelled, and tasted something like the originals, but were becoming more and more the output of a laboratory.

Messaging from health authorities and governments changed significantly, and the message was basically that the new industrially-derived products were healthier than the old fat-laden disaster packages of heart attack and obesity.

On the back of all the chemical advances, supermarkets rose to become the dominant food distribution solution. For the business model of supermarkets to work, production must be centralised, as the sheer number of products required to fill the shelves could never be individually sourced from local, independent producers. Hand in hand with centralised production is a long distribution chain. There are a few things to note here. One, food has to travel a long way to get to your fridge or cupboard. Two, because of the distance the food has to travel, the time between it being produced and you eating it increases when compared with local sourcing. Three, because the food has to appear fresh when you buy it and then eat it, it is more likely to contain chemicals able to perform such a function, and it will often be sealed inside plastic packaging.

Overall, what I am describing is the infiltration of artificial chemicals into every stage of the food cycle, from the growing of it to the processing of it, then the distribution of it, and finally the consuming of it. Even when cooking food, non-stick cookware is the norm. This is made possible by a group of chemicals known as forever chemicals, and these are now accepted to be toxins of great concern(*).

It is very easy to switch to cast iron cookware. Cast iron pans have to be seasoned to make them non-stick, but there is no need to use Teflon for cooking. Cast iron cookware is scientifically shown to provide dietary iron, as well as not being poisonous. The internet has plenty of options for buying cast iron cookware, and plenty of instructions for seasoning a cast iron pan.

The world of science claims all of its inputs into food are great and there is nothing to worry about, but the nutrients that we eat food for are kind of side-lined by it. Even mainstream research is now telling us about a range of common deficiencies across populations. This is presented as an ongoing conundrum, something to spend ever more research money on. If, like myself, you are not a scientist, you will be quickly dismissed if you bring up the methods involved in getting food onto tables.

Chemicals have also found their way into almost all personal hygiene products, along with a vast array of household cleaning products, and are now known to leach out of the plastics we use to package everything up in. Some amount of these products are ingested, breathed in, or absorbed through our skin.

All nutrients, meaning proteins, fats, carbohydrates, fibre (if it can be classed as a nutrient), vitamins, and minerals, have recommended daily allowances assigned to them. Typically, these figures represent either a minimum or maximum amount required to not develop a condition directly related to going outside of those defined boundaries. The numbers have no capacity for adjustment. This allows no scope for a situation where somebody could do with considerably more nutrients to repair some underlying damage.

As an example, most animals synthesise their own Vitamin C. Humans, some apes, and guinea pigs are among the exceptions to this, meaning they have to acquire it from diet alone. As humans, we are told we need somewhere around fifty milligrams of Vitamin C each day, no more, and no less. This figure is, I think, the amount required by a healthy person to prevent scurvy from developing. Now then, Vitamin C, as well as being an antioxidant, is an essential precursor to collagen, so without Vitamin C we cannot produce collagen. Collagen is required to repair damage to cellular structures in the body. So, regardless of whether we have damage to repair or not, we are told we need no more than about fifty milligrams of Vitamin C each day.

Other animals synthesise a great deal more Vitamin C than

our recommended fifty milligrams, with quantities measured in grams, not milligrams, when adjusted for body weight. Animals capable of living in more extreme environments tend to produce relatively more Vitamin C than others. So a rat will produce up to an equivalent of twenty or thirty grams, and a rat can live in a sewer. A goat can produce more Vitamin C than any other animal, apparently up to an equivalent of one hundred grams per day. Goats don't suffer much illness, and if they do become ill they will generally only become ill with something so bad it will kill them outright. They don't get sniffles like us humans do.

Even though we are told we only need a microscopic amount, there is some level of collective knowledge about the healing properties of Vitamin C, and many of us will turn to it when we catch a cold or flu. Probably not enough to have a real effect though, as we are led to believe there is an upper safety limit, somewhere around 1 gram daily, and this is not enough to have much impact on a cold or a flu..

There are likely plenty more times when increased levels of any nutrient would be most beneficial, but we are conditioned into believing that as long as we meet our minimum requirements, then food has little else to offer.

As an example, I go through times when I crave salt. This is most of the time, actually, one of the quirks of having a colostomy. Not the one-dimensional table salt containing sodium and little else other than potential cyanide poisoning, but proper Himalayan rock salt, which has no anti-caking agents, and lots of other minerals in addition to sodium. This is my body telling me it needs one or more of the minerals in the salt. Similarly, I might crave meat, fat, or eggs, and nothing else at certain times, and at other times I want sugar.

Going back to modern food production, the nutrients we need are very much secondary to the business requirements of numerous multinational corporations, and these corporations all lead back to the chemical industry. While we do hear some disjointed stories of how some chemicals are perhaps not all that good, we never get anything like a full picture of how much our lives have been infiltrated by them. This is because the corporations who provide such products, absolutely require the chemicals to be there to have a viable business model. If the full picture of the devastation being wreaked on the environment and the health of people were seriously looked into, those corporations could no longer continue to exist, and we would have no option but to return to a more natural, localised economy. Such an economy would not need the input of the corporations, but the nature of power is such that they are going to do whatever they can to maintain their existence.

Hence the endless scratching of heads regarding the origins of modern disease. There are various diseases, Crohn's included, that simply did not exist in the past. If you apply some deductive reasoning, the addition of chemicals to every area of life must surely be one of the top contenders for what is allowing these new diseases to develop.

Pharmaceutical medicine is another branch of the chemical industry. It is quite interesting to consider that one branch of this industry is providing our sustenance, and a second branch of the same industry is offering the solutions to the problems that I would say are arising out of the first branch, along with additional solutions to the problems it is causing itself. Such a state of affairs is unlikely to ever solve anything, instead causing more of the very same problems it is claiming to be the solution for.

I think there is a very strong case to argue, which is that people such as myself are the canaries in the coal mine of the chemical industry. Just in case you don't know what this means, back when coal mining was still a good thing, canaries were used to detect a build-up of gas underground. Canaries are little colourful songbirds, a bit like budgies, or maybe you could describe them as travel parrots. If the canary suddenly stopped singing and became silent, this was an indication that it was being poisoned by an increase in the amount of gas in the air. The workers would take this as their cue to either get out of the mine or to put respirators on (the canaries were kept in special cages that could pump oxygen in, to revive them). Anyone with an inflammatory condition might well be the canary of modern civilisation and its reliance on chemicals.

So there is my theory of my disease, as best as I can convey it. The origin of it, in my opinion, has something to do with all of the toxic chemicals in the modern world, along with something to do with my psychological profile, and maybe also something to do with things that happened before I was born. I honestly don't think it is either possible or necessary to get the cause of it down to anything more specific than that. The solution is incredibly straightforward and simply involves avoiding a very long list of things that aggravate it.

I started my chapter about my food choices by saying I wasn't going to provide you with a specific diet plan, and I'm sticking with that because you are unique. Also, it is important to follow what your body is asking for, and a fixed meal plan isn't the way to achieve this. However, the things I eat do have some commonality with several mainstream, and not so mainstream, diets, so you might want to investigate some of them. If you do, then here are a few ideas to get you started.

First of all is the FODMAP diet. FODMAP stands for Fermentable Oligosaccharides, Disaccharides, Monosaccharides And Polyols. It is one of the few diets that recognises soluble fibre as potentially being a problem and suggests meal ideas that minimise exposure to such things.

There is also a Specific Carbohydrate Diet, which is claimed to offer good results for Inflammatory Bowel Disease, and has similarities with the FODMAP diet.

Next is the Paleo Diet. This takes the approach of eating the kinds of things we would have eaten before modern society came about, so foods that would have been available to hunter-gatherers. This is heavily focused on meat and eggs but does include fruits and vegetables. The general theory behind the Paleo Diet is to remove the processed elements of modern diets.

The Keto Diet is kind of similar to Paleo, but is more focused on the elimination of carbohydrates, thus forcing the body to burn fat for energy. Probably not the best idea if you have a disease that makes you underweight, giving you a lack of body fat to begin with.

A more extreme version of these last two is the Carnivore Diet, which is similar, but eliminates all plant-based foods.

None of these diets are entirely suitable for me, but you might find one or other of them, or elements from them, to be of some benefit.

One subject that is rearing its head at the moment is Ultra Processed Food, and the dietary choices I have made do seem to align with the basic premise that the production of food, the processing of it, and the adding of artificial ingredients to it, is becoming a major issue in the modern world. So a bit of reading up about this might be of great benefit.

Other than that, if you have a disease similar to the one I've spent so much time with, then my experience suggests that if you want to be rid of it, then there is a route out. You have to find your road map, though. All that I, or anyone else, can do, is point you in the right direction, but at least I will admit this. Be very wary of anyone offering you an all-encompassing solution, especially if it involves you paying them for it. Also, don't expect to find immediate answers in the endless range of food and nutritional supplements on offer. It is probably better to find and remove whatever is causing the problem before adding something else into the mix.

I have never heard anyone claim that Crohn's disease, at least once you have it, is related to the microscopic, indigestible parts of food, while I have heard almost every other theory imaginable. My original motivation for writing this was to show that the solutions on offer were the cause of more of the very same problems, and I hope to have done just that, even if just in some small way. The medical industry openly admits it does not know what causes Crohn's, and as such, it cannot claim to have any reasonable idea about how to resolve it. This lack of understanding is just what is needed for treatments that ultimately make your health worse.

If you are looking for a way to get on top of Inflammatory Bowel disease, you have nothing to lose by trying an interpretation of the things I have outlined, apart from maybe needing to find a bit of extra cash for your weekly shopping. You will know very quickly whether it works, so you can decide whether to stick with it, or you can go back to whatever you are doing now. If you do try though, you need to go all-in on it. Avoiding just one or two things at a time won't show any positive results.

My perspective on Crohn's is that once you have it, it can be a short-lived, temporary illness, albeit a rather acute one.

Unfortunately, the medical system, as far as I see it, makes the disease a very serious, unrelenting, unending one. To add to this, most accepted nutritional advice is potentially missing the point, and as such might also be helping to perpetuate it. The changes in dietary habits I have identified, become, quite literally, the very things you are least likely to consider.

I'm going to finish with two questions, which have the same answer. Just before I do that, if you have made it here then thank you for reading the book. I genuinely hope you have gained something from it, even if that is just some different perspectives to think about. If you feel others might benefit from it, or even just derive some entertainment, then please consider leaving a review.

OK then, question 1: In terms of medicine, it isn't as if the standard treatments are just a little bit off the mark. It could be argued that the way Crohn's and similar diseases are treated, is as far removed as it is possible to be from anything that would fix the problem. How is it that the medical industry can have its approach to such diseases so badly wrong?

Question 2: How was it that I just went along with the treatments on offer for a long, long time, and didn't begin to seriously consider there might be a better option, even though all the evidence I needed was right in front of me all along?

The answer to both questions is faith in the structures of society, or put more simply, believing what someone else is saying. For myself, I felt I was in no position to question the experts, as I thought they were the keepers of the best information. Those experts imparted knowledge taken on faith from a range of other experts, built on top of many previous iterations of the very same process, something that allows for an ever-increasing accumulation of mistakes, with no way of being able to identify, or even acknowledge the existence of those mistakes.

We tend to equate complexity with progress, so will often patch over and around erroneous thinking, rather than just go back to basics and rethink something. We do this personally, within family and social groups, and even right up at the level of society as a whole. As such, we are prone to dismiss the simple, and often glaringly obvious answers.

About the Author

Kevin Kendall is a resilient individual who has triumphed over serious, long-term illness, emerging stronger and more determined than ever. Originally a self-taught computer games programmer, his journey has taken an artistic turn, where he now expresses his creativity as a visual artist.

Kevin's most significant accomplishment is his unwavering spirit in the face of adversity. Battling and overcoming a serious, long-term illness has not only shaped his character but has become a testament to his strength and tenacity.

A lifelong learner, Kevin seeks to unravel the mysteries of human belief. His curiosity drives him to explore and understand the intricacies of what makes people believe the things they do.

You can connect with me on:
- https://www.kevink2.co.uk
- https://twitter.com/northeastheret1